Slimming with the Hay Diet

by Ursula Summ

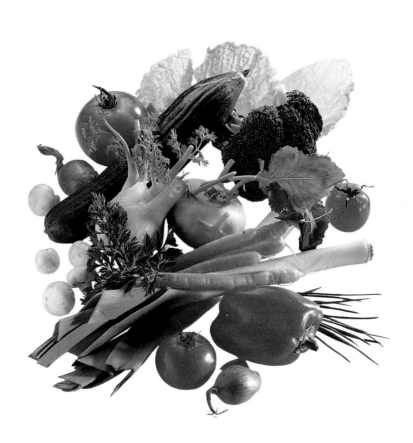

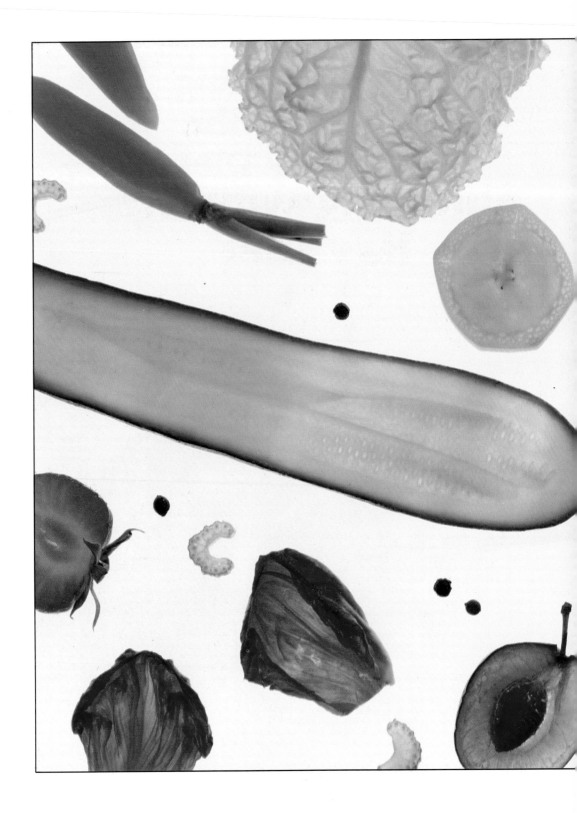

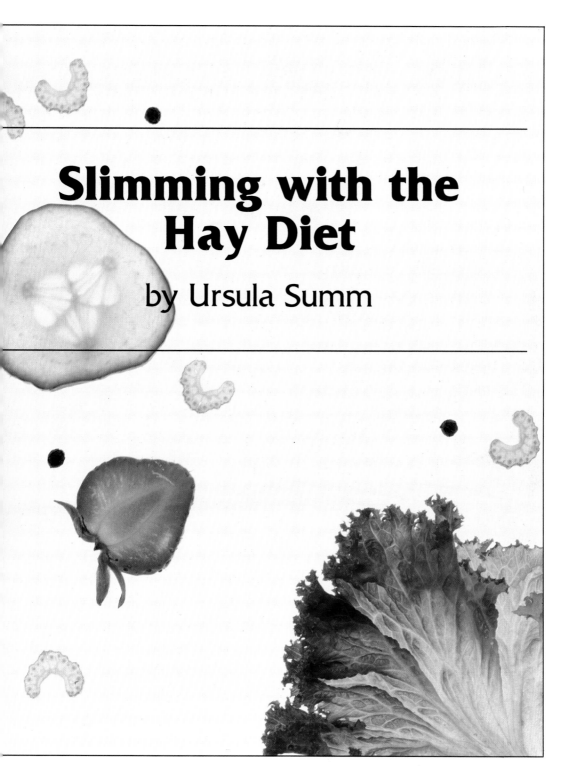

Slimming with the Hay Diet

by Ursula Summ

foulsham
LONDON • NEW YORK • TORONTO • SYDNEY

foulsham

The Publishing House
Bennetts Close, Cippenham, Berks SL1 5AP

ISBN 0-572-02043-0

Originally published by Falken-Verlag GmbH,
Niedernhausen TS, Germany.
Photographs copyright © Falken-Verlag

Editor: Birgit Wenderoth

Production: Albert Brühl
Title Picture: TLC Foto Studio GmbH, Velen Ramsdorf
Photos: TLC Foto Studio GmbH, Velen Ramsdorf;
p.9: A 63 Schilling & Schmitz, Cologne;
p.29 bottom: Fotostudio Wolfgang Feiler, Karlsruhe;
p.2/3, 23 and 24: Brigitte Harms, Hamburg;
p29 centre: Studio Margit Schwarz, Frankfurt;
p.26/27 and 34/35: Michael Wissing, Waldkirch
Drawing: Gerhard Scholz, Dornburg.

The advice in this book has been carefully considered and checked,
however, no responsibility can be taken.

Responsibility of the author and publishers and employees for
persons and material damage will not be accepted.

Phototypeset in Great Britain by Typesetting Solutions, Slough, Berks.
Printed in Great Britain at Cambus Litho, East Kilbride

CONTENTS

Foreword

Because of my heavy work schedule, it is not now possible for me to take on as much lecturing and teach-in commitments as I used to and therefore I have written this book as a substitute. It is designed specifically for working people with limited time who want to lose weight healthily, and contains many tips on how to implement food combining in a relaxed, easy-to-follow and personal manner without disrupting a busy day in the work place.

There has recently been considerable rethinking in the field of safe and sensible dieting and many slimmers in general, and doctors and nutritionists in particular, have come to the conclusion that gimmicky and crash course diets can be hazardous to health and rarely bring about the desired and permanent weight loss expected. This is where the Hay diet comes into its own.

Invented by American Dr Howard Hay just before and during World War I, food combining is a cleverly conceived and flexible concept in which slimmers can diet more or less as they please without having to conform to a rigid regime. The good news is that it works, it is essentially practical and regarded by dieters as an undemanding godsend.

Hay's food combining system is not a slimming diet as such, but rather a way of blending foods harmoniously together so that they don't shout at each other. The end result? The body gets rid of unwanted toxins and, simultaneously, combats over-acidity. This increases vitality and produces a pleasing sense of well-being. The side effect is a natural and lasting weight loss.

Additionally, Hay's system does not scream expenditure and esoteric ingredients which need searching out. YOU choose whether you want your food to be economically-priced; middle-of-the-road or costly; simple or heading towards a touch of luxury; plain or fancy. This makes menu-planning easy and enables you to eat a little – or a lot – of what you fancy at home, while away on business trips or abroad on holiday.

As actions speak louder than words, try food combining for yourself and then evaluate the long-term benefits, mentally, spiritually and physically.

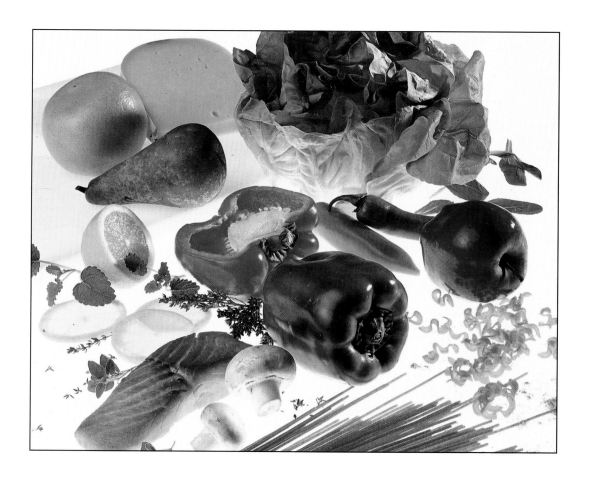

What Are the Causes of Overweight?

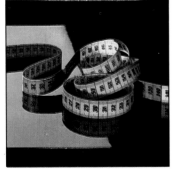

Do We Eat the Wrong Things?

There are basically two types of overweight people. There are those with smallish appetites who are perpetually active yet never lose any weight despite how little they eat or how often they diet. Then there are others who admit to eating too much, especially fatty and sugary foods, and tend to be couch potatoes. The thought of physical exercise is enough to make them reach for the crisp packet, then along comes vanity or a warning from the GP and they go on yet another diet. Neither group succeeds in losing weight. Why?

Jumping from diet to diet could be one reason because the body is subjected to a start-stop situation which upsets the metabolic balance and gets the person nowhere, least of all slim. Another reason could be semi-starvation, the 'lose weight at any price' attitude when people reduce their food intake drastically and then console themselves with extra cups of tea or coffee, the odd nibble, a cigarette. Often this leads to an almost uncontrollable desire to consume excessive amounts of chocolate, cakes, sweets, biscuits, crisps and other snack foods which turn out to be nothing more than quick fixes. Healthwise, this all adds up to poor nutrition which can cause dizziness, headaches, fatigue, depression and a susceptibility to illness.

What Is to Be Done?

One this is certain: there is no such thing as a miracle diet and starving the body of food does not help the overweight. It is better to take a much more relaxed approach. Find out the reason for eating. Is it really hunger, or do you just fancy it? Do you eat out of frustration or boredom? Try to recognise the pitfalls when out shopping. Advertising should not be underestimated either, as it penetrates our subconscious mind more than we realise.

Learn to understand the faults in your own eating habits and try to change your routine and outlook. Looking young and slim and striving to keep that way may not be right for YOU, your genes or your personality. Give yourself a realistic weight target then set about achieving it little by little without expecting overnight miracles. If you lose weight slowly, about 200 to 300 grammes (7 to 11 oz) a week, you are far LESS likely to put it on again in a hurry. And remember, with food combining you can enjoy the odd indulgence without coming to any harm – a piece of chocolate when you crave something sweet or a few salted nuts if you fancy a savoury.

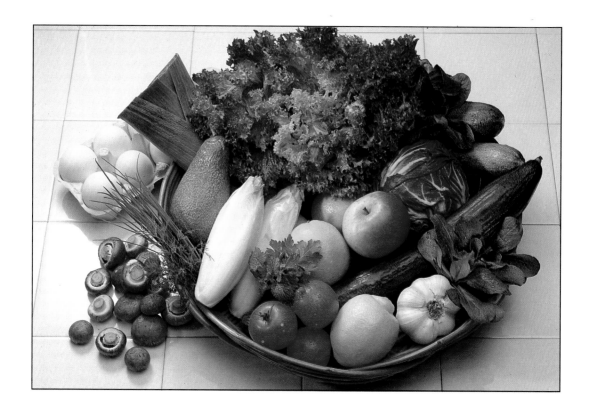

Are Our Eating Habits Wrong?

Do you ever feel bloated and heavy after eating a meal in a hurry, and has it ever occurred to you that there is a possible link between hasty eating and overweight? Relaxed mealtimes, in a pleasant atmosphere, will do wonders for the digestion and enable you to metabolise food properly and thus reduce flatulence, indigestion and discomfort. Always eat slowly, avoid arguments round the table and getting up more than is absolutely necessary during the meal.

Do you analyse your eating habits? Do you pay heed to the quality of your nutrition or are you interested only in what things taste like? Do you eat very little during the day then make up for it by eating twice as much in the evening? Do you chew your food properly or just gulp it down automatically, not much caring what you eat as long as you fill up on something? Do you eat quickly and greedily and then feel guilty? Does any of this register? It should, because thousands and thousands of people are becoming unconsciously and unnecessarily overweight through careless eating and, in the process, becoming more and more unhealthy.

What Is to Be Done?

Think about what you eat at every mealtime. Increase your intake of natural foods like cereals, potatoes, brown rice, vegetables (fresh or frozen) and fresh fruit and salads. Reduce the amount of flesh foods you eat. Learn to eat calmly' and in an atmosphere of quiet. Chew slowly so that enzymes in the saliva can begin the process of digestion as soon as the food reaches your mouth. If you habitually bypass the action of chewing, it will result in indigestion.

Is Being Too Heavy Due to Psychological Reasons?

The idea that the cause of overweight lies in the area of the psyche is inadequately recognised.

Have you ever asked yourself what your relationship is with your body? Do you like every part of yourself or do you take a negative stance? Do you reject yourself because, for example, your legs are too fat or your hips appear to you to be too broad? Has this view of yourself fixed itself so firmly in your consciousness that you give your body no other opportunity but to become even fatter? Do you have these negative thoughts because you do not look as you would like?

Thoughts have tremendous energy. The power of thought can lead to self-enslavement and weakness which can bring about much suffering in consequence, as all mental suggestions eventually turn into reality. Your body becomes a stage and often represents what you think. And as you think yourself fat, your subconscious mind turns this into reality. Make it a daily habit to observe your thoughts, as we are all subject to the laws of suggestion. Help yourself to success by taking control over your thoughts. Master your weakness of thinking negatively and become enthused with positive powers that unfold from within you. Recognise the power of thought and the power of feelings. If you try to cast aside worries and troubles, carry unsolved problems around with you, have to

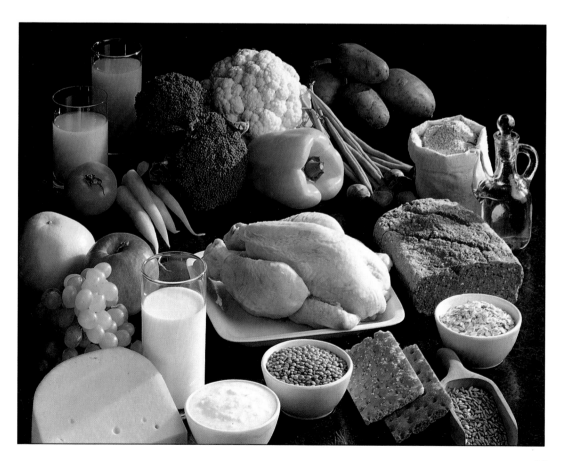

fight with professional or private difficulties or are simply dissatisfied, then your body will soon lose its psychological balance. Your overweight is then an attempt by your body to draw attention to personal problems.

If you want to change anything you must begin with yourself. Do you eat because you are fearful; do you suffer from loneliness, or are you in urgent need of protection? Perhaps one of these causes lies buried in your subconscious from childhood. Did you always have to clear your plate? Were you given sweets when you felt lonely? Do you reward yourself in a similar way now when you are cross, bored, tired or depressed?

Only you can answer these questions, but to adopt a negative attitude would be a waste. From now on you have to plan for the future instead of delving into the past and take positive steps to help yourself. Only in this way will you be able to relieve psychological tensions and pressure.

Relaxation Works Wonders

Begin by learning to relax and let go of everything that depresses you. Strive to be happy, peaceable and calm. Take an imaginary trip every day which will take up only a few moments of your time. The following exercise can be carried out without professional guidance: sit down on a comfortable chair, hold your back straight and breathe evenly and quietly. Close your eyes and relax. Take leave of your problems without hesitation or regret. As you release psychological tension your head will become clear, the spirit free, the soul more finely tuned. Your body's battery will be recharged. Every time you exercise, your heart will seem lighter.

Dr Hay's Food Combining

The human body is a complex biochemical factory with its own set of rules. Break them, and you are asking for trouble, healthwise and weightwise.

Dr Hay developed food combining in order to combat his own serious kidney complaint after he was seemingly beyond conventional medical help. For a long time he tried to analyse his own illness. He looked into the chemical combination of the human body and discovered that it consisted of up to 80 per cent alkaline elements and up to 20 per cent acid elements. He also took note of the incompatibility of individual foodstuffs with each other, as he knew that protein breaks down only in an acid solution, and carbohydrates in an alkaline solution. Accordingly, he put together his daily food plan, eating largely alkaline and less acid foods. He also separated those with a high carbohydrate content from those high in protein. Food combining was born and Dr Hay cured.

What is Distinctive about Food Combining?

The main characteristic, as the name indicates, is combining foods in a particular way. Within a meal, foods containing mainly carbohydrates are separated from those containing mainly protein and eaten separately. Naturally, complete separation is not possible and is therefore not attempted. The idea and purpose of separating foods in this way is to harmonise them with each other in order to avoid excess strain on the digestive system.

Many of you will doubtless have already discovered that a higgledy-piggledy mixture of foods at mealtimes causes indigestion. But did you know it can ultimately lead to obesity and lethargy?

Briefly, we shall follow the route of food through the body. First is the mouth and the most important stage of digestion takes place here where the salivary glands release and distribute the enzyme amylopsin which pre-digests carbohydrates. Carbohydrates are present in large quantities in cereals, bread, noodles, potatoes and rice.

The second stage of digestion takes place in the stomach. Here the proteins are pre-digested with the help of the hydrochloric acid and the digestive enzyme pepsin. They are broken down into smaller constituents. Protein is found in large quantities in meat, fish, cheese, eggs and milk.

According to Dr Hay, it is against digestive principles to eat protein and carbohydrate together. His reason for this is simple; consumption of protein starts off the production of hydrochloric acid and pepsin in the stomach, but these juices hinder the working of the amylopsin from the saliva. If we eat only carbohydrates then only small quantities of acid juices will be produced in the stomach and the amylopsin will be more effective. Carbohydrates can then be better digested.

The third stage of digestion takes place in the upper part of the colon, the duodenum. This is where the pancreas becomes active whose enzymes, together with the gall coming from the liver, perform numerous functions. The pancreas is made up of two parts. In one part the hormones insulin and glycogen are produced and pass into the blood as required to regulate blood sugar. In the other part, digestive enzymes are produced; trypsin and chymotrypsin (enzymes that break up protein), amylopsin (enzymes that break up carbohydrates) as well as lipase (an enzyme that breaks down fat). Without these enzymes no digestion can take place in the small intestine.

In order to ensure that the complex process of digestion is unproblematic, the pancreas should be underworked. This means not indulging in excessive amounts of food at one sitting because even the best can become a burden, remain only partly digested and lead to flatulence.

Through the villus of the intestines and subsequently through the blood and the lymph, the broken-down and digested food, together with vitamins and minerals, move to the liver where they are utilised as required by the body.

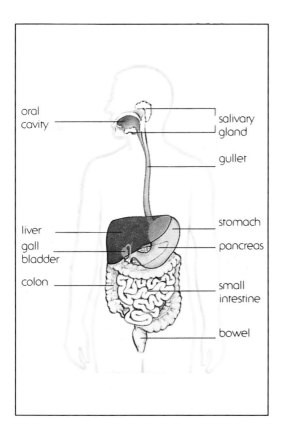

oral cavity

salivary gland

gullet

liver

gall bladder

colon

stomach

pancreas

small intestine

bowel

The Food Combining Principle of Dr Hay

Food combining means harmonising different foods to bring order into the digestive system. Combining is not at all difficult, once you understand what it is about and have mastered the technique. The food combining plan on pages 18 and 19 tells you exactly which foods belong to the protein group (printed in blue) and which fall into the carbohydrate group (printed in red). In a further group there are neutral foods (printed in black).

The neutral foods can basically be mixed in a meal with foods from the protein as well as the carbohydrate group. Some of the foods you should eat sparingly. Amongst these are butter and meat, sausages and ham, and generally anything smoked or pickled. Such foods will also be found in the combining plan, but this does not mean you can eat as much as you fancy. Opt for small portions.

'Neutral', for the purposes of food combining, means that these particular items and foods will not disrupt either the digestion of proteins or carbohydrates. They harmonise with all foods. You may find some things about this arrangement contradictory, but it is based on many years' experience. For example, soured milk products, though full of protein, are listed as neutral, as the protein has been changed in the souring and is therefore easier to digest. Raw meat or raw fish are also protein-rich foods, but are additionally listed as neutral because their cell structure has not been changed. If heated they will be affected so that the changed protein becomes more difficult to digest.

All fats are neutral and cover cold pressed and naturally produced oils, butter and cream, full-fat cheese (from 60 per cent fat), smoked fish and raw sausage products. Fats are not digested in the stomach but in the duodenum, and therefore do not interfere with the digestive process. Dr Hay calls this form of diet 'food separation'. This has led to some confusion world-wide as it is not possible to separate completely proteins from carbohydrates. The term 'food combining' was therefore thought more suitable.

What Do We Mean by Over-acidity?

The acid–alkaline balance is another important factor in Hay's food combining. According to Dr Hay, an adequate consumption of alkaline-producing foods is essential to good health.

On the other side are the acids. Every day the human organism is confronted by acids in the body which are brought about by the digestive processes. Here we are talking about uric acid, carbonic acid and lactic acid, just to mention a few. At the same time, many alkaline elements are also produced. Our bodies can survive only if there is a satisfactory balance of acid and alkali in the blood and tissues and fortunately we have a built-in buffer system which does the job for us. However, food eaten under stress can produce acidity with unpleasant side-effects.

According to Dr Hay, many protein-rich and carbohydrate foods are acid-producing. For example, meat, sausages, eggs, cheese and different carbohydrates such as sugar, processed cereals and white rice. Vegetables, salads, seed sprouts and fruit belong to the alkaline producers. The minerals, vitamins and fibre they contain make a decisive contribution to sound metabolism and one should ensure that meals comprise approximately 20 per cent of acid-producing foods and 80 per cent of alkaline-producing foods, raw whenever possible as in salads and fresh fruit.

Suggestion for a protein meal:
1 part meat, fish, eggs or cheese (e.g. 100 g or 3½ oz) to 3 to 4 parts vegetables and salads, cooked or uncooked (respectively 300 to 400 g, 11 to 14 oz).

Suggestion for a carbohydrate meal:
1 part potatoes, natural rice, wholemeal noodles or cereals (e.g. 100 g or 3½ oz) to 3 to 4 parts vegetables and salads, cooked or uncooked (respectively 300 to 400 g, 11 to 14 oz).

It is not only through the consumption of food that acids are produced in our bodies. Permanent psychological pressure, e.g. as a result of family or professional stress, noise, shock or fear, can cause a rapid increase in the acid balance. Thus a healthy and calm life style is beneficial all round.
Here are a few additional tips for a healthy, balanced diet:
Acid-rich fruit such as berries, stone and core fruit and citrus should never be eaten with foods belonging to the carbohydrate group. It is best to eat these only in small amounts with foods from the protein group, or eat them as a treat for breakfast, as a snack between meals, or enjoy them on hot days as a complete midday meal.

After 3 o'clock in the afternoon, it is recommended that fruit (except for bananas, cranberries and dried fruit) should not be eaten as it can cause fermentation and subsequent flatulence.
Apples play a special role in food combining. Fresh apples belong to the group of acid-rich fruit. Freshly harvested, they contain large amounts of fruit acid and therefore belong to the protein group.
A soft, sweet apple has less acid, but contains a higher amount of carbohydrate. It can also therefore be mixed with cereals, wholemeal noodles, pasta, natural rice or potatoes within a meal (such as apple cake, apple compôte with rice or pasta or as muesli with grated apples).

Wholefood Food Combining

It is proven that health and well-being is, to a large extent, dependent on a good diet and the proper provision of nutrients, vitamins, minerals and fibre. Unfortunately, our present day Western diet is made up of white flour products, ready-made products, animal products with hidden fats and salt, as well as sweet foods, puddings, biscuits and ice cream – all highly processed and therefore containing only a few valuable ingredients. For this reason many nutritionists recommend a wholefood diet comprising salads, vegetables, potatoes, fruit, wholemeal cereals and products made from them, natural rice and cold pressed oils. When combined with protein foods (minimal amounts) we are giving our bodies adequate nutrition.

It is advisable to follow a wholefood diet slowly at first to prevent flatulence and discomfort in the gut. The intestines must first learn how to digest food properly again. Cereals and wholegrain products with a high proportion of roughage (as well as raw food) can lead to problems for those with sensitive intestines. If you are one of these people, you should first try out which vegetables suit you best when eaten raw, and those which you need to steam until just tender.

Sprouts and shoots are real little vitamin bombs. These can be obtained in well-stocked stores, in wholefood shops or you can grow them yourself.

In a balanced, wholefood diet, it is essential to drink adequate liquids. Water has a large number of tasks to perform and one of its major roles is to assist digestion and distribution of nutrients. The best method of maintaining the balance of liquids in the body is to drink sufficient fluids in the form of herb or fruit tea, as well as mineral water. One can generally take it that an adult requires 2 to 3 litres (3½ to 5 pints) of liquid per day – whether thirsty or not. In healthy food combining, the meals should contain only 1 to 1½ litres (1¾ to 2½ pints) of liquid (in fruit, vegetables, salads and raw food), as these foods contain an average of 80 to 90 per cent of water.

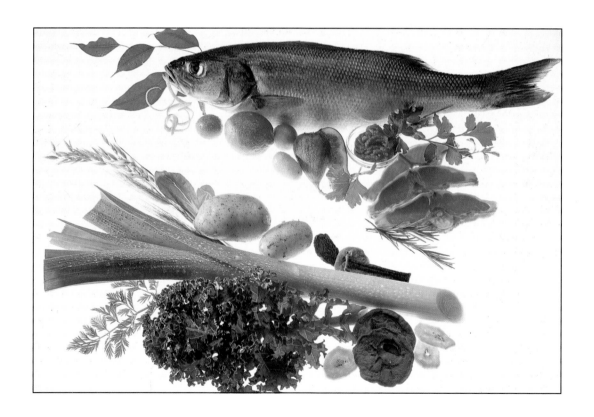

Within one meal, food belonging to the protein group should *not* be mixed with those from the carbohydrate group. The following combinations are possible:

● Food from the protein and the neutral group.

● Food from the carbohydrate and the neutral group.

Protein Group

All types of cooked meat

This includes e.g.:

Beef: roast, stewed, braised, steak, minced meat dishes, burgers.

Veal: escalopes, stewed or roast.

Lamb: cutlets, back, leg, shoulder.

Pork is not recommended.

All kinds of cooked poultry meat. For example, goose, duck and chicken.

All kinds of cooked sausage and meats. For example, fried sausages, liver sausage, corned beef, boiled ham and poultry sausage (pork sausage and salami are not recommended, but many kinds of sausage are available without any pork content).

All kinds of non-smoked, cooked fish as well as cooked shellfish and crustacea. For example, plaice, cod, salmon, tuna, mackerel, halibut, herring, trout, mussels, prawns, lobster and crab.

All soy products. For example, tofu, soy sauce as well as sandwich spreads made of soya.

Eggs

Milk of all fat levels

All kinds of cheese with a maximum of 50 per cent fat. For example, Parmesan, Emmenthal, Edam, Gouda.

Cooked or canned tomatoes

Drinks. For example, fruit tea, apple wine, dry white and red wine, sparkling wine.

All berry fruits. Except cranberries.

All cored fruit. Except soft, sweet apples.

Stone and citrus fruits

All exotic fruit. Except bananas. For example, mangos, papayas, kiwis, melons. (Dr Hay places acid-rich types of fruit in the protein group. However, in my own groups, it has been shown that only small amounts of these fruits should be eaten with other foods from the protein group. Or eat this type of fruit with milk or soured milk products for breakfast or in between meals.)

Tip:

Do not use breadcrumbs to coat food from the protein group, but sesame seeds, ground almonds or nuts instead.

Neutral Group

Neutral foods can be mixed in the same meal with protein as well as carbohydrate.

All fats. For example, oil (cold pressed preferable), unhardened margarine types with a high content of polyunsaturated fatty acids, butter, white vegetable fat.

All soured milk products. For example, quark, yoghurt, kefir, thick soured cream, soured cream and buttermilk.

Cream and coffee cream

All kinds of cheese with at least 60 per cent fat. For example, double cream soft cheese, Gouda, Brie, Camembert, Cheddar, Stilton, Parmesan.

All kinds of white cheese. For example, sheep's and goat's cheese, Mozzarella, cottage cheese.

All raw, smoked types of sausage and meat. For example, smoked meat, raw ham, salami, blood sausage (all obtainable without pork).

Raw meat. To be avoided.

All types of raw, marinated or smoked fish. For example, smoked salmon, smoked halibut, kippers, eel, mackerel, trout, rollmops.

The following vegetables: Aubergines, artichokes, broccoli, cauliflower, green beans, green peas, fennel, cucumber, garlic, kohlrabi, leek, sweetcorn, carrots, (bell) peppers, radishes, horseradish, beetroot (red beet), sprouts, red cabbage, sauerkraut, celery, asparagus, spinach, tomatoes, white cabbage, Savoy cabbage, onions, courgettes (zucchini), all leaf salad (also iceberg, endive, corn salad), chicory (endive) and Chinese cabbage as well as all varieties of mushroom.

All sprouts and shoots

All herbs and spices

All nuts and seeds (apart from ground nuts). For example, hazel nuts, coconut chips, almonds, sesame seeds.

Bilberries

Raisins

Olives

Egg yolk

Yeast

High alcohol percent spirits. For example, Schnaps and Juniper brandy.

Herb teas

All gelatine products. For example, gelatine (animal product), agar agar (a powdered seaweed – the powder is dissolved in cold liquid, it is all then heated to 60–80°C and left to cool), vegetable thickening made from carob (health shops).

Tips:
Dressings for salads that are to be eaten with protein meals should be made from oil, cream, herbs and lemon juice. Dressings to be eaten with carbohydrate meals should be made from soured milk products such as kefir, thick soured milk and yoghurt.

Carbohydrate Group

All kinds of cereals. For example, wheat, rye, barley, oats, millet, sweet corn, brown rice.

Buckwheat

All kinds of wholemeal cereal products. For example, wholemeal bread and bread rolls, cakes from wholemeal flour, wholemeal pasta, wholemeal semolina.

The following types of vegetables and fruit: Potatoes, kale, salsify, bananas, untreated dried fruit (except raisins – they are neutral; currants on the other hand belong to the carbohydrates), fresh dates and figs and soft, sweet apples.

The following sweeteners: Frutilose, honey, maple syrup, pears and thick apple syrup.

Various products: Potato flour, cream of tartar, custard powder, carob.

Beer

Tip:
Cereal rissoles should be coated only in wholemeal breadcrumbs, ground nuts or sesame seeds and not previously turned in egg.

Please avoid:

White flour and all products made from it. For example, sweet and savoury biscuits as well as pasta and polished rice.

Sugar, sweeteners and products made from them. For example, sweets and jams, ready-made meals and conserves.

Dried pulses. For example, peas, lentils, beans.

Ground nuts

Cranberries

Pork and all pork products

Raw meat

Uncooked egg whites

Ready-made mayonnaise

Vinegar

Hardened fats. For example, normal types of margarine and hard, white frying fats.

Black tea, coffee, cocoa and high percent spirits

You can, if you like, avoid these foods altogether. Those suffering from kidney complaints should avoid consuming large quantities of spinach, rhubarb, chestnuts, horseradish, mustard and pepper.

Generally, you should eat as little meat as possible. This is also true for everything smoked (neutral) and pickled (carbohydrate), as they may contain substances which cause cancer. It is up to you to choose.

Watch your salt consumption. Too much salt is unhealthy. Sausages, cheese, ready-made meals and some breads are high in salt and should be eaten cautiously.

Quantity Plan

The quantities and time of meals on the quantity plan are approximate guides only and you should adapt them to suit your own convenience.

Starving and fasting are pointless. No-one should leave the table hungry, because the inevitable snacking between meals will result.

But always remember: To remain healthy everyone's body needs sufficient vegetables, salads and fruit, which should be eaten in part raw.

1 glass (about 200 ml/7 fl oz) low-carbonated mineral water.

Breakfast

One has the choice between a carbohydrate, a protein or a fruit meal.

Carbohydrate meal

1 slice wholemeal bread (50 g/2 oz)
or 1 wholemeal bread roll
or 3 slices wholemeal crispbread
  spread thinly with butter or margarine and eaten with:
  30 g/1¼ oz sausage (approx. 3 slices)
or 30 g/1¼ oz cheese of 60 per cent fat (approx 1 slice)
or 50 g/2 oz quark (approx. 2 dessertspoons)
or 10 ml/2 tsp honey
as an alternative:
muesli or a cereal porridge (see page 36).

Protein meal

2 eggs (fried, scrambled, boiled or poached) (More than 3 eggs per week is not recommended). Accompanied by: tomatoes, cucumbers, peppers, radishes or another neutral vegetable, but *no* bread.

Fruit meal

Plenty of fresh seasonal fruit, except bananas, figs and dates.

Anyone who wants to drink tea or coffee should add to it a little cream or honey.

Important. Chew every bite very carefully and mix well with saliva. Coffee or tea is no substitute for saliva.

1 large glass fruit or herb tea or still mineral water.

1 large glass fruit or herb tea or still mineral water.

Break

200 g/7 oz seasonal fruit (but no bananas, figs and dates)
or 250 ml/8 fl oz fresh milk
or 250 g/8 fl oz soured milk product
or 100 g/4 oz fruit (but no bananas, figs and dates) accompanied by 120 ml/4 fl oz milk or soured milk products

1 large glass fruit or herb tea or still mineral water.

Midday Meal

For lunch one can choose between a protein or a carbohydrate meal.

Protein meal

100–150 g/4-5 oz meat
or 150–200 g/5-7 oz fish
or 2 eggs
or 60 g/2½ oz cheese up to 50 per cent fat
or 80 g/3 oz cooked sausage, accompanied by 400 g/4 oz neutral vegetables and/or salad

Carbohydrate meal

50 g/2 oz cereal (weighed uncooked)
or 50 g/2 oz natural rice (weighed uncooked)
or 50 g/2 oz wholemeal pasta (weighed uncooked)
or 200 g/7 oz cooked potatoes accompanied by:
400 g/4 oz vegetables or salad

25–50 g of neutral foods can be eaten with these (see Combining Plan on pages 18–19).

In addition to the ingredients for the protein or carbohydrate meals, small amounts of butter, margarine, oil or cream can be used. They are all neutral and go well.

During a main meal nothing should be drunk. If you do need to have a drink, sip it slowly.

1 large glass fruit or herb tea or still mineral water

1 large glass fruit or herb tea or still mineral water

1 large glass fruit or herb tea or still mineral water

Break

1 banana
or 1 muesli bar without sugar
or 1 piece of cake (see pages 46 and 48)
or 2–3 biscuits (see pages 49 and 50)
or 1 slice crispbread with honey
or 1 tbsp quark with 1 tsp honey
or ½ tbsp wholemeal oat flakes and carton yoghurt
or 200 g/7 oz soured milk products

Drink no fresh milk, as it is more difficult to digest in the afternoon.

1 large glass fruit or herb tea or still mineral water.

Evening meal

In the evening one has the choice of a carbohydrate meal

50 g/2 oz cereals (weighed uncooked)
or 100 g/3½ oz wholemeal bread
or 50 g/2 oz natural rice (weighed uncooked)
or 50 g/2 oz wholemeal pasta (uncooked weight)
or 200 g/7 oz cooked potatoes accompanied by:
400 g/14 oz vegetables and salad, 25–50 g/1–2 oz neutral foods and a small amount butter, margarine, oil or cream

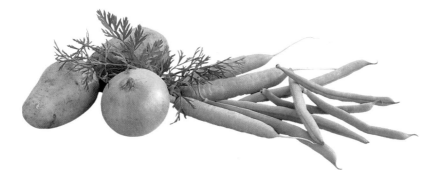

Food Combining in Practice

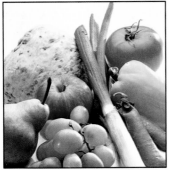

Changing to a Food Combining Diet

Before changing over to food combining, it is essential to have a changeover day. This serves to stimulate the metabolism and helps in elimination of toxins. Choose between a vegetable-salad day, a fruit day, a potato drink day and a potato-vegetable-soup day.

You should, in addition, drink plenty of liquids in the form of tea (such as fruit tea) or still mineral water. Except on the fruit day, you may have a LIGHT breakfast. The following will explain what is meant by a clearing-out day, and you can choose the one you prefer for yourself.

Vegetable-salad Day
Eat only vegetables in season, uncooked or lightly steamed, and/or salad. Add neither fat nor salt. If required, a little vegetarian vegetable broth (instant powder) can be used. Eat any quantity of vegetables you fancy, but obviously within reason.

Fruit Day
Eat fresh fruit until 3 o'clock (but please no bananas, fresh figs or dates), in any quantity you wish. Follow at 5 o'clock with two medium-sized bananas and/or 2 medium-sized potatoes, cooked in their skins.

Potato-drink Day
This form of clear-out is recommended for all those with sensitive stomachs and intestines. Cook 500 g/18 oz of washed, unpeeled potatoes in 2 litres/3½ pints of water (without salt). Eat the skins of new potatoes but peel mature ones. Purée potatoes with the cooking liquor and drink this at intervals throughout the day.

Potato-vegetable-soup Day

This soup is made of 3 potatoes, 3 onions, 3 leeks, 1 small celeriac and (according to taste) 3 carrots. The exact weight of the ingredients does not matter. Clean the vegetables, wash and dice. Place in a large saucepan and fill with water. Add fresh or dried herbs and spices (caraway, garlic, parsley, marjoram, lovage), but add no salt. Cook until vegetables are soft. The soup, if you prefer, can be seasoned with vegetarian vegetable broth (instant powder). Reheat and eat at intervals through the day.

Tips for People at Work

Is it possible to go out to work, have little spare time and, despite this, still eat a balanced diet consisting of good, healthy food? Yes, assuming that you are prepared to change your eating habits somewhat. Once you really want to change, then the possibility of permanent success is very real indeed. Put stress on hold, be patient with yourself if you get irritable and avoid snacking. Above all, never eat foods you positively dislike. The food combining diet gives you plenty of choice so always opt for what you enjoy.

Please remember that **enemy number 1** for the overweight is hurry. Hasty eating at home, or eating on the hoof, make for indigestion. Eat in a leisurely way, even if it takes a few minutes more.

Enemy number 2 is lethargy. The causes are manifold but take-away meals eaten on the hop are not always sustaining and lead to fatigue if consumed on a regular basis. No matter how simple, a freshly-prepared meal will do you more good than anything you can buy. If you are too pressed for time to cook, eat fruit and vegetable meals.

Enemy number 3 is the fact that we forget about ourselves due to pressure of work and do not prepare the next meal ahead of time. Suddenly we become hungry, everything edible is in the freezer so we reach for a snack, often loaded with calories.

Enemy number 4 is our indifference towards what we eat. 'I'll settle for anything' is not designed to keep you trim, slim and healthy. Always choose cautiously.

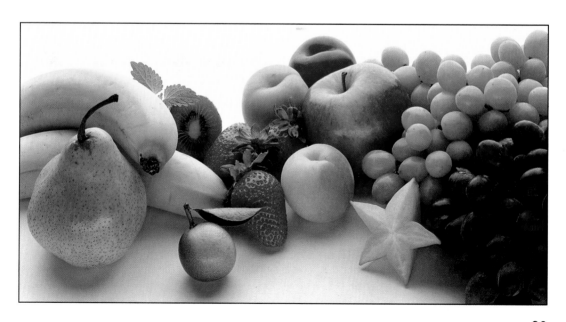

Enemy number 5 is a heavy main meal in the evening. The digestive system has to fight to cope towards the end of the day and it doesn't take too kindly to an overload of food. You are best to keep the evening meal light to prevent discomfort and also an increase in weight.

A realistic diet change could look like this:

Breakfast
Eat a generous slice of wholemeal bread, a bowl of muesli or some fresh fruit instead of white rolls or white toast.

Your bread can be spread thinly with butter and then topped with a slice or two of sausage or cheese, from 60 per cent fat. Allow about 25–30 g/1 oz or so.

The simplest breakfast of all is fruit. Throughout the morning you can eat as much seasonal fruit as you like. Bananas, fresh figs and dates should not be eaten with sharp fruit. These three types belong to the carbohydrate group and so do not go well with sour fruits.

If you do not want to go without your coffee or tea, take it with a little coffee cream, perhaps sweetening it with some honey.

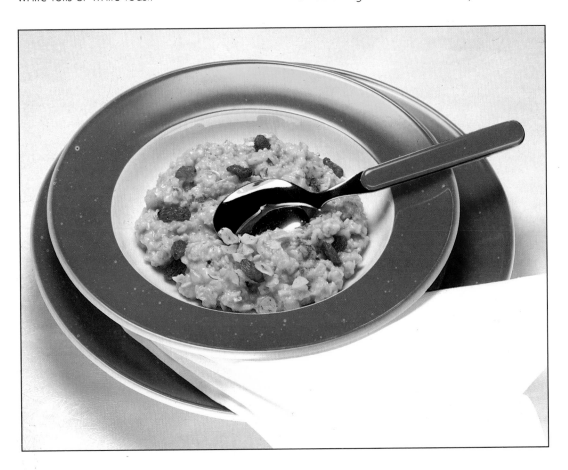

In the Morning

Too little sugar can be just as harmful to the system as too much. Therefore have a mid-morning snack of fruit or fresh vegetables to include apples, pineapple, oranges, carrots, fennel, kohlrabi, cucumber or tomatoes.

Mid-day Meal

Choice 1: eating in the canteen

If you are fortunate enough to have a good canteen at your place of work, you should use it, observing a few simple rules. In a canteen, as in a restaurant, it is usual for meat, fish and egg dishes to be on offer. In addition there will also be potatoes, rice, pasta, salad or vegetables. As the menu for the complete week is usually known in advance, you can plan ahead to suit yourself. Tick off everything you would like to eat and decide whether you want a protein or a carbohydrate meal. With the help of the combining plan on pages 18 and 19, you can check out whether the meal follows the general rules of food combining. Should the salad or vegetable portions be insufficient, you should bring some from home to top up. Perhaps the cook will be prepared to come to some arrangement with you whereby the meat or potatoes are changed for more salad or vegetables. Should there be something on the menu which does not conform strictly to the principles of food combining, but is one of your favourite dishes, you can indulge yourself with a good conscience from time to time without feeling guilty.

Choice 2: take your own food

This is an alternative when there is no canteen at work, or you do not want to use it. In order to save time and energy, I recommend that you prepare the meal the day before (recipe two portions) at 1½ times the quantity. During the previous evening you can eat two portions with your partner, eating the rest yourself the following midday. Should your partner or a colleague, perhaps, like to eat something cooked at lunchtime, then double quantities can be prepared so that there is sufficient for the next day.

Do you have a microwave or mini-oven at work? If so, prepared meals can be warmed-up just before eating. Salads can be prepared the previous evening or, if you have time, in the morning. Pack the salad ingredients and dressing in separate containers and mix them together immediately before eating to prevent the greenery from wilting. Another tip: prepare the salad sauce at home in a large quantity (see pages 92–95). It can then be kept in a screw-top jar for several days in a refrigerator. This way you will save time and have a tasty salad dressing readily available. Mixed drinks or desserts can also be prepared easily at home and transported to work in airtight containers. In the weekly plans on pages 28-31 you will find many suggestions for meals to take to work.

By the way: potatoes, rice and pasta are easy to cook in large portions. For example, potatoes boiled in their skins in the evening can be used in a potato salad the next day. Rice can be prepared sweet or savoury; even pasta can be prepared in various ways to suit taste: with garlic and a little olive oil, with mushroom sauce, as baked pasta or as a salad.

The same is true of vegetables and carrots, green beans, cauliflower, kohlrabi as well as white and red cabbage can all be prepared in large quantities. As all these types belong to neutral foods they can be used with protein as well as with carbohydrate meals. For a protein meal, for example, the vegetables can be combined with roast beef, cold roast lamb, cold chicken, eggs and cheese (low-fat types) as well as with fried or boiled fish.

Choice 3: eating in a restaurant

If you go to eat in a restaurant, you should decide beforehand whether you want to eat a protein or carbohydrate meal. Should you be uncertain about what foods belong in what group, take this book along with you. With the help of the food combining plan on pages 18 to 19 you can then plan a meal, perhaps enlisting the help of the waiter.

Should you decide on a protein meal ie meat, fish or eggs, accompany with a double portion of salad or vegetables instead of the more customary potatoes, rice or pasta.

Example:
    1 steak with 1 double portion salad
or salad selection with roast chicken or turkey (no potatoes)
or ½ chicken with plenty of green salad
or roast meat with gravy, 1 double portion of vegetables
or steamed or grilled fish, such as trout, 1 salmon steak or a large fillet of plaice with a generous salad or 1 double portion of vegetables .
or 1 omelette, scrambled egg or 2 fried eggs with 1 large salad

If you would prefer a carbohydrate meal, choose potatoes, rice or pasta and have alongside a choice from the neutrals:
    a portion of cheese like Brie, Camembert or Stilton
or slices of Parma ham or salami
or smoked fish such as salmon, mackerel or trout fillets. Gravadlax (marinated salmon). Rollmops.
Order a large mixed salad besides or a selection of assorted vegetables.

About 20 minutes before your midday meal, munch some fresh fruit or raw vegetables like carrots. It will reduce your appetite and additionally aid digestion.

Afternoons

In the afternoon the blood sugar level drops considerably in most people and a snack is advisable. Have a few dates, dried figs or 1 medium ripe banana.

Evening meal

Keep it light, choosing carbohydrates with plenty of fresh vegetables and/or salad. There are some interesting recipe ideas for potatoes, rice and pasta on pages 59–73.

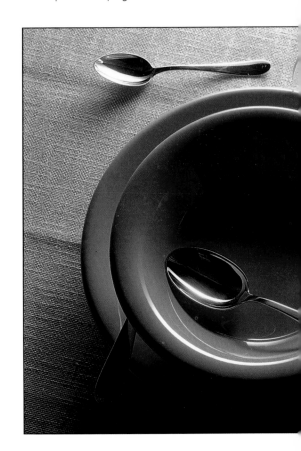

Weekly plans

Here are two weekly plans, especially designed for working people which are equally useful for holidays or times when you are at home. Plan 1 is for fairly fast meals; Plan 2 for times when you have to cook.

The amounts for evenings, and for midday and evenings meals at the weekend (Saturday and Sunday) are sufficient for two portions. Should you be catering just for yourself, reduce the quantities accordingly. All other dishes are designed for one portion.

Always remember that it is important to drink sufficient between meals (see pages 20–21).

Notes and ideas for your own Hay Diet

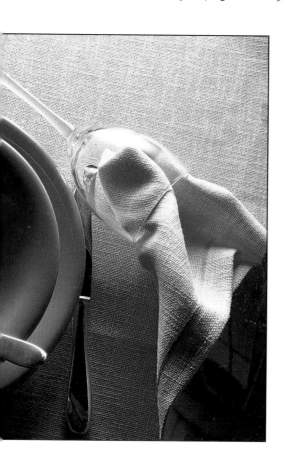

Weekly Plan 1

	Breakfast	Snack
1st day (Monday)	Every day choose from: fresh fruit (except bananas, figs and dates) *or* 1 slice wholegrain bread spread thinly with butter with 30 g/1½ oz cheese (60 per cent fat) or 30 g/1½ oz turkey roll *or* 1 bowl of muesli or ceral porridge (page 36)	Every day choose from: 200 g/7 oz fresh fruit (except bananas, figs and dates) *or* 200 g/7 oz neutral raw food
2nd day (Tuesday)		
3rd day (Wednesday)		
4th day (Thursday)		
5th day (Friday)		
6th day (Saturday)		
7th day (Sunday)		

Midday meal	Snack	Evening meal
1 wholemeal roll, plus 1 carton (150 g/5 oz yoghurt (3.5 per cent fat) and 2 young carrots	Every day a choice of: 1 banana _or_ 1 sweet apple _or_ 150 g/5 oz buttermilk _or_ yoghurt	Spaghetti with garlic sauce (page 65), plus a plate of raw food
200 g/7 oz cottage cheese plus 2 slices wholemeal crispbread and 1 small cucumber (peeled, cut into slices)		Oyster mushroom ragout (page 71), plus 100 g/4 oz (raw weight) brown rice, cooked
1 wholemeal roll, plus 100 g/4 oz Mozzarella, 3 beef tomatoes sprinkled with chopped basil		Courgette (zucchini) soup (page 57), plus 1 wholemeal roll per portion
2 boiled eggs, plus 1 large pepper		Curry pot (page 73)
1 wholemeal roll, plus 400 g/14 oz raw sauerkraut and 250 ml/8 fl oz buttermilk		Tagliatellli with vegetable and cheese sauce (page 66)
Boiled potatoes with tsatsiki (page 68); cook double amount of potatoes and keep half the potatoes for next day		Piquant filled pancakes (page 70)
1 portion grilled chicken (remove fatty parts), plus 450 g/1 lb green beans, cooked and tossed in 2 tsp butter		Using the potatoes from yesterday, make Potato and celeriac salad (page 61)

Weekly Plan 2

	Breakfast	Snack
1st day (Monday)	Grape picker's breakfast (page 40)	1 orange
2nd day (Tuesday)	Fruity quark (page 40); Sauce and 1 portion vegetables for the raw food plate (page 52)	200 g/7 oz fresh fruit (except bananas, figs and dates)
3rd day (Wednesday)	Wholemeal bread with cottage cheese and walnuts (page 40); Mixed farm salad (page 77); prepared grapefruit yoghurt (page 44)	Grapefruit yoghurt (page 44)
4th day (Thursday)	Apple muesli (page 36)	1 generous portion of water melon
5th day (Friday)	Quark bread (page 38), salad and sauce	2 carrots
6th day (Saturday)	Oat flake muesli with baked prunes (page 36)	1 mango
7th day (Sunday)	Sweet porridge (page 36)	1 apple Loaf tin cake with apple pieces (page 48)

Midday meal	Snack	Evening meal
150 g/5 oz carton yoghurt (3.5 per cent fat), 1 wholemeal roll and 1 small cucumber	2 wholemeal crispbreads spread thinly with butter and honey	Cheesey toasted bread roll (page 61), plus Lambs' lettuce with celeriac and tofu (page 55) 1 portion from the Raw vegetable platter (page 52)
Raw vegetable platter (page 52)	150 g/5 oz carton yoghurt (3.5 per cent fat)	Filled oven potatoes (page 67) Prepare Mixed farm salad (page 77) (pack sauce and salad separately)
Mixed farm salad (page 77)	1 sweet apple	Carrot soup (page 58) and Mushroom and millet risotto (page 72)
1 wholemeal roll with 1½ tbsp double cream soft cheese, plus 150 g/5 oz fresh vegetables	1 banana	Wholemeal baguette with piquant sauerkraut salad (page 62); prepare Endive and orange salad (page 55) (pack sauce and salad separately)
Endive and orange salad (page 55)	1 muesli bar without sugar	Savoury potato salad (page 61); Soak prunes for the Oat flake muesli (page 36)
Italian minced meat fry (page 79)	Buttermilk drink (page 44)	Pan pizza (page 68)
Fillet of beef with leek (page 80)	1 piece Loaf tin cake with apple pieces (page 48); the rest of the cake can be deep frozen	Spaghetti with courgette (zucchini) (page 65)

Eating on Holiday

Even on holiday one can eat well and still follow Dr Hay's rules of food combining. Do not book full board as it is easier if you can cater for yourself. Alternatively, choose bed and breakfast packages.

In hot climates a fruit meal will often be sufficient at lunchtime. As the main meal of the day is normally eaten in the evening, start with a large plate of salad followed by a smallish portion of meat, fish or poultry. If you can avoid eating late, so much the better.

Valuable Tips for Food Combining

• Never eat food from the carbohydrate and protein groups together (see plan pages 18–19).
• Eat as naturally as possible. Avoid commercial processed foods, ready-made meals and foods with a long sell-by date.
• It is preferable to eat raw or lightly cooked raw vegetables, salads, potato dishes and wholemeal products.
• Avoid sweet things, such as sweets, chocolates, chocolate bars and sweet biscuits made of white flour. Instead of using sugar to sweeten, opt for honey, thick fruit juice, raisins and dried fruit. Although high in calories, they also contain important vitamins, minerals and fibre. Even so, use sparingly.
• Do not add too much salt and ready-made seasonings to your food. It is better to use fresh or dried herbs instead.
• Use lemon juice instead of vinegar for salad dressings.
• Untreated, cold pressed oils, unhardened fats, butter, cream and eggs (in small quantities) provide valuable materials the body cannot make for itself.
• Drink a glass of mineral water, herb or fruit tea in between meals to stave off hunger pangs.

• Do not skip meals. If you really are not hungry, eat a little fresh fruit or vegetables.
• Plan your meals in advance and never go shopping on an empty stomach as temptation might get the better of you.
• Chew your food well, and mix it well with saliva. Try not to drink anything during meals.
• To cook with minimal fat, aluminium foil is ideal for parceling up food for baking. All it needs is a light brush over with melted butter or margarine.

Hints on the Recipes

• All the recipes in this book are easy to cook and should provide you with good examples of how protein, carbohydrate and neutral foods can be combined.
• So that the arrangement of the recipes into the three groups is easy to follow, the **recipe names** are printed in different colours.

red   =   carbohydrate meal
blue   =   protein meal
black =   neutral meal

• In every recipe the number of portions is stated. If you want to make more or less, adjust quantities accordingly.
• The quoted *kilocalories (kcal) and kilojoules (kj)* refer to 1 portion or 1 piece.
• The *ingredient quantities* refer generally to uncooked and uncleaned foods.
• The *preparation times* in the recipes include preparation time (washing, cleaning, cutting), as well as the cooking or baking time. These are approximate. Special times such as soaking, leaving to rise or to cool, are given as extras.
• If you wish to vary a recipe in some way or develop your own, please use the combining plan on pages 18 and 19 to assist.
• For those members of the family who do not wish to join in food combining, it is not necessary to cook especially for them. Add meat or fish to the carbohydrate meals and potatoes, rice or pasta to protein meals.

• Some of the recipes use ingredients obtainable only in health food shops.

Vegetable thickening agents such as carob seed flour have no taste and contain few calories. Use the powder sparingly, as it thickens quickly. Please take special note of the instructions for use on the packet.

I very strongly recommend the use of **sea salt**, as it contains important essential minerals and vitamins, such as iodine.

Also **herb salt** (its cooking salt content is about 84 per cent) as it is excellent for adding flavour.

Vegetarian vegetable stock is good for sprinkling (instant powder) and is produced by a number of manufacturers. It is made only of vegetable ingredients and so is free of cholesterol. It is also gluten-free and contains no hardened fats.

Baking powder. Make up your own baking powder using 2 parts cream of tartar to 1 part bicarbonate of soda. It will then be free of additives.

Natural rice is unepeeled rice. In contrast to polished white rice, it contains a lot of fibre and is therefore recommended. In recipes, it is always soaked overnight so that its relatively long cooking time is shortened. It can also be cooked without soaking for 35 to 45 minutes.

• In Food Combining, the choice and proper use of **oils and fats** is important. Recommended are natural, untreated, cold pressed, unrefined oils that contain polyunsaturated fatty acids. Olive, sunflower, thistle, wheat germ, linseed and corn oil are available in this quality. Try to use only olive or sunflower oil, as both can be heated satisfactorily without damage to themselves.

Butter and unhardened vegetable fats are made with a high proportion of polyunsaturated fatty acids and are also recommended. As they are high in calories, they should be used only in small quantities. They should not be overheated or cooked until brown.

Not recommended are hardened fats such as normal margarine or hard white fat recommended for frying. Avoid refined oils, such as normal salad oil.

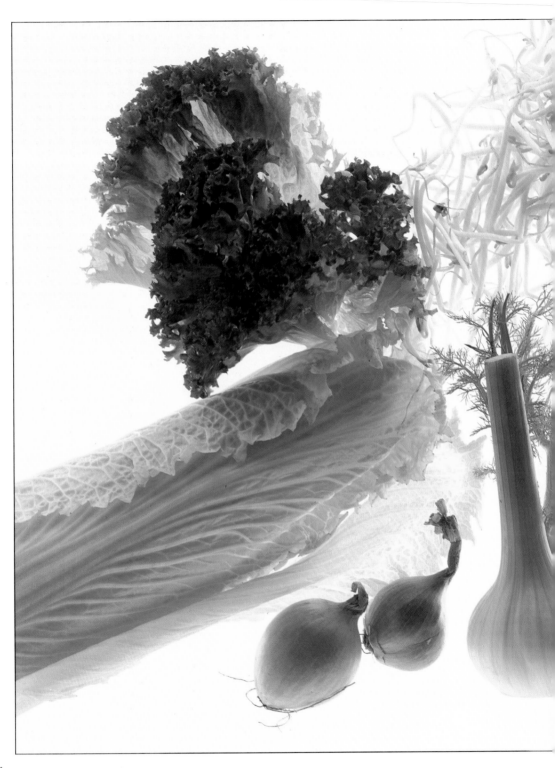

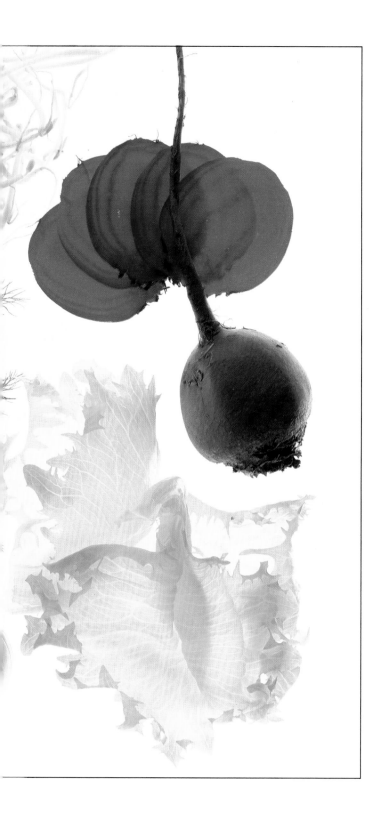

The
Recipes

Ideas for Breakfast

APPLE MUESLI

Preparation time: 15 minutes

Serves 1

1 eating apple
120 ml/4 fl oz/½ cup yoghurt, 3.5 per cent fat
10 ml/2 tsp glucose
20 ml/1½ tbsp rolled oat flakes

1. Wash the apple, quarter, remove the core and grate coarsely.

2. Mix the yoghurt with the glucose until smooth then mix in the grated apple.

3. Tip the oat flakes in a bowl and pour on the yoghurt mixture.

about 300 kcal/1255 kJ

Photograph opposite (second from top)

BANANA YOGHURT

Preparation time: 10 minutes

Serves 1

1 small banana
150 ml/¼ pt/⅔ cup yoghurt, 3.5 per cent fat
10 ml/2 tsp sunflower seeds

1. Peel the banana and crush with a fork.

2. Lightly whisk the yoghurt until creamy then stir in the banana purée. Sprinkle with sunflower seeds.

about 225 kcal/940 kJ

Photograph opposite (second from bottom)

SWEET PORRIDGE

Preparation time: 10 minutes

Serves 1

50 g/2 oz rolled oats
300 ml/½ pt/1¼ cups water
15 ml/1 tbsp whipping cream
10 ml/2 tsp honey
a pinch of ground cinnamon

1. Crush the oats with a rolling pin. Put into saucepan.

2. Add the water and cream. Slowly bring to the boil, stirring continuously.

3. Sweeten lightly with honey and sprinkle with cinnamon.

about 330 kcal/1380 kJ

Photograph opposite (top)

OAT FLAKE MUESLI WITH PRUNES

Soaking time: approx 8 hours or overnight
Preparation time: 10 minutes

Serves 1

3 prunes
20 ml/1½ tbsp oat flakes or rolled oats
120 ml/4 fl oz/½ cup Greek-style yoghurt
5 ml/1 tsp honey
a pinch of ground cinnamon

1. Leave the prunes to soak in water overnight.

2. Before eating, cut the prunes into small pieces. Mix with oat flakes, yoghurt and some of the soaking water.

3. Sweeten the muesli lightly with honey and sprinkle with cinnamon.

about 290 kcal/1210 kJ

Photograph opposite (centre)

FRENCH SOFT CHEESE BREAD

Preparation time: 10 minutes

Serves 1

50 g/2 oz full-fat cream cheese
15 ml/1 tbsp mineral water
1 clove garlic
2–3 basil leaves
2.5 ml/½ tsp herb salt
1 slice wholemeal bread

1. Lightly whip cream cheese with the mineral water until creamy. Peel and crush garlic clove and add.

2. Wash the basil leaves and chop finely. Add to the cheese with the herb salt. Mix well.

3. Spread wholemeal bread with cheese mixture.

about 300 kcal/1255 kJ

Photograph opposite (bottom)

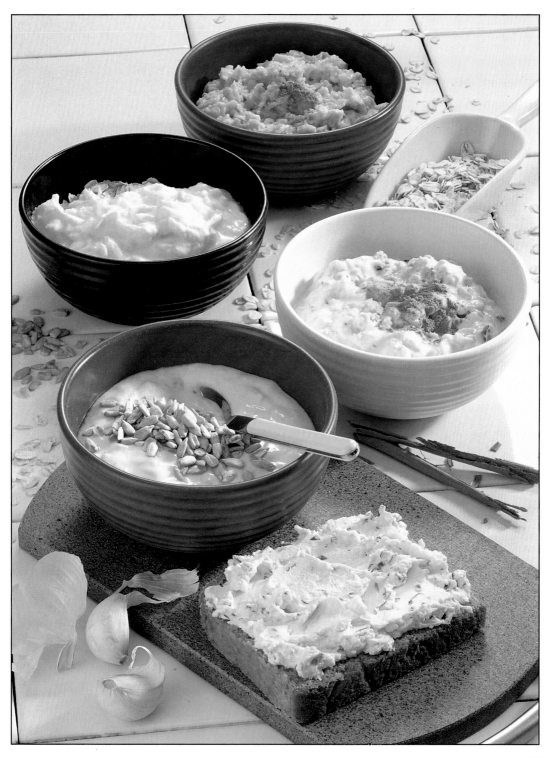

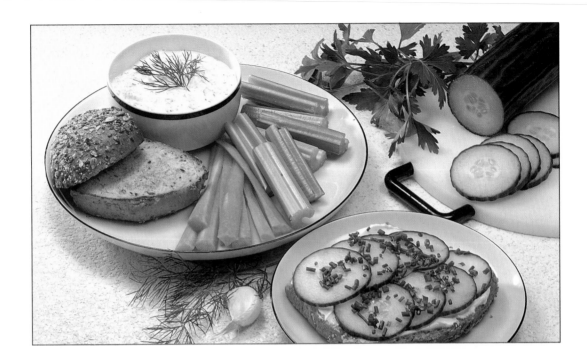

WHOLEMEAL BREAD ROLLS WITH PIQUANT HERB CREAM

Preparation time: 15 minutes

Serves 1

For the cream:

100 gl/4 oz quark, 20 per cent fat	
120 ml/4 fl oz/½ cup yoghurt	
20 ml/1½ tbsp chopped fresh herbs (parsley, chives, coriander, dill)	
1 clove garlic, crushed	

In addition:

2 carrots	
3 celery sticks	
1 wholemeal bread roll	

1. Mix the quark with the yoghurt. Stir in the herbs and garlic. Season lightly with sea salt.

2. Clean the carrots, wash, peel and quarter lengthways. Wash the celery sticks.

3. Cut the bread roll in half and toast both halves. Dip the raw vegetables in the herb cream and eat with the wholemeal roll.

about 460 kcal/1925 kJ

Photograph above (left)

Tip:

The herb cream (neutral) goes well with potatoes boiled in their skins or fried potatoes. It is also suitable for spreading on bread.

QUARK BREAD

Preparation time: 10 minutes

Serves 1

75 g/3 oz quark, 20 per cent fat	
15 ml/1 tbsp mineral water	
sea salt	
1 slice wholemeal bread	
5 ml/1 tsp butter	
8 thin slices cucumber	
10 ml/2 tsp chopped fresh chives	

1. Beat the quark with the mineral water until smooth and season with sea salt.

2. Spread the wholemeal bread thinly with butter. Cover with quark.

3. Top with cucumber and sprinkle with chives.

about 240 kcal/1000 kJ

Photograph above (right)

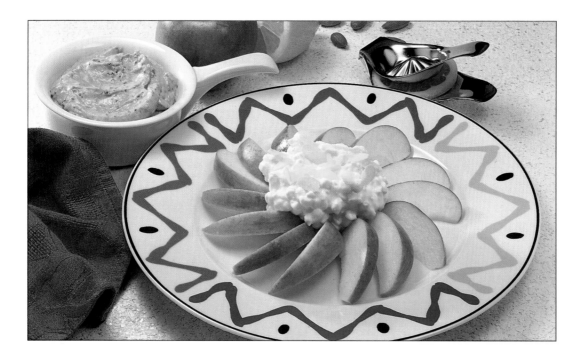

SWEET BREAD SPREAD

Soaking time: approx 8 hours

Preparation time: 15 minutes

Serves 10

200 gl/7 oz prunes
200 ml/7 fl oz water
finely grated rind of 1 lemon
200 g/7 oz full-fat cream cheese
a large pinch of ground cinnamon

1. Leave the prunes to soak in water for 8 hours or overnight.

2. Next day pour the water into a small bowl. Remove the stones from the prunes.

3. Purée prunes until smoothish in a food processor. Add the lemon rind. Thin down to a creamy consistency with the soaking water.

4. Stir in cheese and season with cinnamon.

about 120 kcal/500 kJ

Photograph above (left)

Tip

This sandwich spread can be kept in the refrigerator for 5 to 7 days. It tastes particularly good on wholemeal rusks or crispbread.

COTTAGE CHEESE WITH APPLE SEGMENTS

Preparation time: 10 minutes

Serves 1

1 eating apple
10 ml/2 tsp lemon juice
100 g/4 oz cottage cheese
5 ml/1 tsp flaked almonds

1. Wash the apple, quarter and cut out the core. Cut apple into thin segments and sprinkle with lemon juice.

2. Arrange the cottage cheese and apple segments attractively on a plate. Sprinkle with almonds.

about 190 kcal/795 kJ

Photograph above (right)

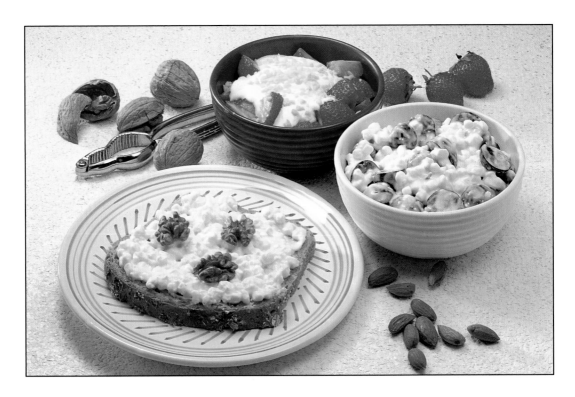

WHOLEMEAL BREAD WITH COTTAGE CHEESE AND WALNUTS

Preparation time: 10 minutes

Serves 1

1 slice wholemeal bread
5 ml/1 tsp butter
75 g/3 oz cottage cheese
3 walnut halves

1. Lightly toast the bread and spread with butter.

2. Break up the cottage cheese with a fork, spread over the bread and sprinkle with walnut kernels.

about 270 kcal/1130 kJ

Photograph above (left)

FRUITY QUARK

Preparation time: 10 minutes

Serves 1

150 g/5 oz strawberries
10 ml/2 tsp golden syrup, melted
100 g/4 oz quark, 20 per cent fat
15 ml/1 tbsp mineral water
10 ml/2 tsp chopped almonds

1. Wash the strawberries. Slice and place in small dishes. Sweeten lightly with the syrup.

2. Stir the quark and mineral water together and spoon over the strawberries. Sprinkle with the almonds.

about 280 kcal/1170 kJ

Photograph above (centre)

GRAPE PICKERS' BREAKFAST

Preparation time: 10 minutes

Serves 1

150 g/5 oz grapes
100 g/4 oz cottage cheese

1. Wash grapes, halve and de-seed.

2. Place the cottage cheese in a small dish and fold in the grapes.

about 210 kcal/880 kJ

Photograph above (right)

Snacks, Desserts and Biscuits ▬▬▬

VANILLA PUDDING WITH BLUEBERRY PURÉE

Preparation time: 15 minutes

Serves 4

150 ml/¼ pt/⅔ cup whipping cream
350 ml/13 fl oz/1½ cups water
30 ml/2 tbsp cornflour
30 ml/2 tbsp golden syrup, melted
a small pinch of ground saffron
1 vanilla pod
300 g/11 oz fresh blueberries
12 fresh mint leaves

1. Combine the cream with the water. Smoothly mix the cornflour with 5 tbsp of cream and water. Stir in the syrup and saffron. Pour into a saucepan.

2. Add the remaining cream and water. Scrape out seeds from the vanilla pod and add.

3. Bring slowly to the boil, whisking all the time, until the mixture thickens.

4. Wash the blueberries and purée two-thirds.

5. Spoon the purée into four small dishes and spoon the cornflour mixture evenly on top. Garnish with mint leaves and the remaining blueberries.

about 240 kcal/1000 kJ

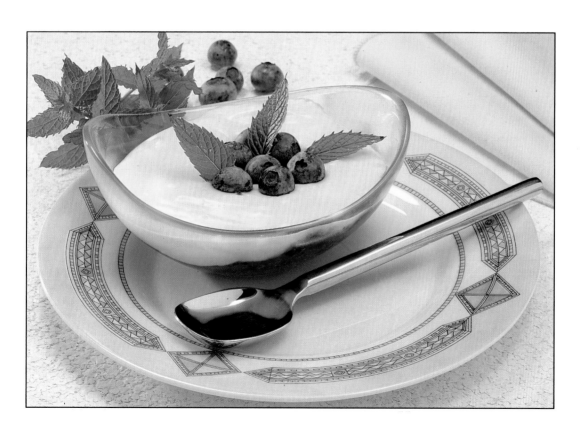

BERRY COCKTAIL WITH RASPBERRY SAUCE

Preparation time: 20 minutes

Serves 2

For the sauce:

250 g/9 oz raspberries
(can be deep-frozen)

15 ml/1 tbsp golden syrup, melted

15 ml/1 tbsp clear raspberry liqueur
(brandy) or Kirsch

For the cocktail:

100 g/4 oz blackberries

100 g/4 oz blackcurrants

100 g/4 oz strawberries

10 ml/2 tsp lemon juice

15 ml/1 tbsp golden syrup, melted

250 g/9 oz quark, 20 per cent fat

30 ml/2 tbsp mineral water

1. To make the sauce, wash the berries then purée in a food processor. Pass through a sieve into a bowl. Mix in the liqueur or Kirsch.

2. To make the cocktail, rinse the berries in a colander under cold running water. Drain well. Tip into a bowl. Add the lemon juice and syrup.

3. Beat the quark with the mineral water until creamy. Spoon into dessert dishes. Place the fruit on top. Coat with raspberry sauce.

about 400 kcal/1675 kJ

Photograph opposite (top)

ORANGE SALAD WITH RUM CREAM

Preparation time: 20 minutes

Serves 2

12 skinned almonds

3 medium-sized oranges

120 ml/4 fl oz/½ cup whipping cream

15 ml/1 tbsp rum

1. Coarsely chop the almonds.

2. Peel the oranges, removing all the white pith. Cut out the orange segments with a sharp knife and arrange in a ring on a plate.

3. Beat the cream until stiff and stir in the rum.

4. Spoon or pipe the rum cream on top of the oranges. Sprinkle with the almonds.

about 330 kcal/1380 kJ

Photograph opposite (bottom)

BLACKBERRY CREAM

Preparation time: 10 minutes
Soaking time: 30 minutes
Setting time: 1 hour

Serves 2

For the sauce:

250 g/9 oz blackberries

30 ml/2 tbsp golden syrup, melted

10 ml/2 tsp gin

10 ml/2 tsp gelatine

30 ml/2 tbsp cold water

175 ml/6 fl oz/¾ cup creamy milk

10 ml/2 tsp flaked almonds

1. Wash the blackberries, crush with a fork, sweeten with syrup and leave to stand for about 30 minutes until juice begins to run.

2. Purée with the gin in a food processor.

3. Soak the gelatine for 5 minutes in water then melt in a saucepan over a low heat. Gradually stir into the blackberry purée.

4. Stir the milk smoothly into the blackberry/gelatine mixture.

5. Spoon into dessert dishes, sprinkle with almonds and set in the refrigerator for about 1 hour.

about 320 kcal/1340 kJ

Photograph opposite (centre)

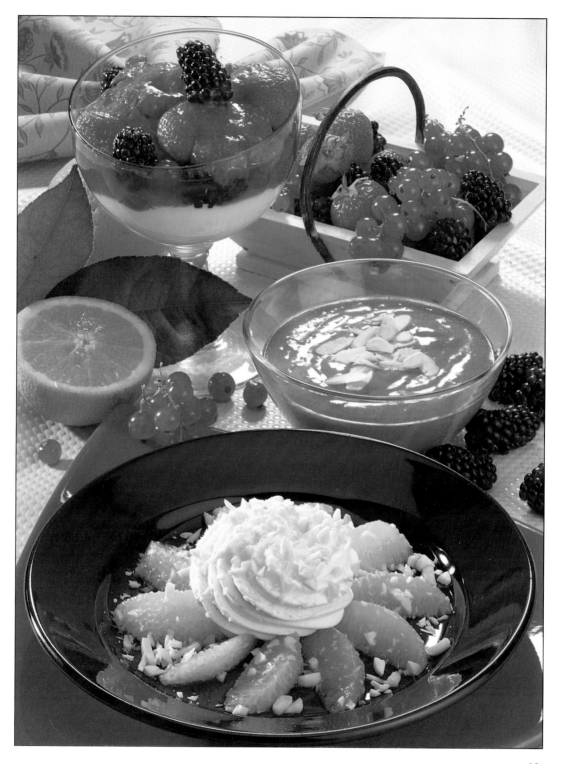

BUTTERMILK DRINK

Preparation time: 10 minutes

Serves 2

2 blood oranges
1 mango
350 ml/12 fl oz/1½ cups buttermilk, chilled
10 ml/2 tsp golden syrup

1. Halve and squeeze out the juice from the oranges.

2. Peel the mango and cut away the flesh from the stone.

3. Purée the orange juice, mango flesh, buttermilk and syrup together in a food processor until smooth.

4. Pour into tall tumblers.

about 210 kcal/880 kJ

Photograph (top)

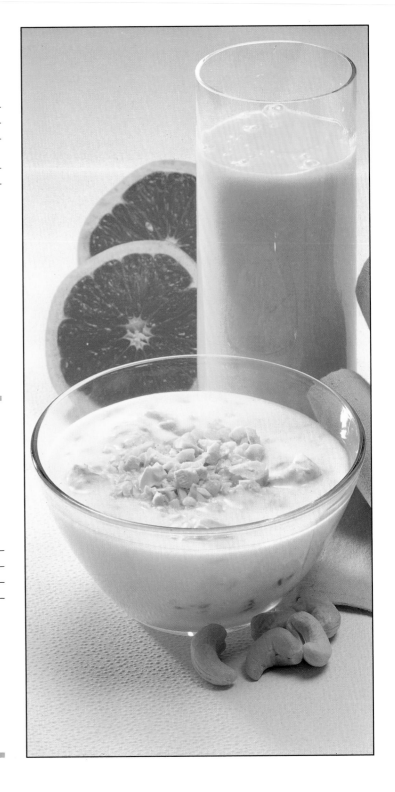

GRAPEFRUIT YOGHURT

Preparation time: 10 minutes

Serves 2

2 pink grapefruit
300 ml/½ pt/1¼ cups yoghurt
30 ml/2 tbsp chopped cashew nuts

1. Peel the grapefruit and remove the pith. Cut the flesh into small pieces.

2. Mix the cubes with the yoghurt. Pour into dishes and sprinkle with the cashew nuts.

about 335 kcal/1485 kJ

Photograph (bottom)

RASPBERRY ICE CREAM

Preparation time: 20 minutes

Freezing time: 2–3 hours

Serves 2

250 g/9 oz raspberries
150 ml/¼ pt/⅔ cup water
15 ml/1 tbsp golden syrup
2 egg yolks
75 ml/5 tbsp whipping (heavy) cream
150 ml/¼ pt/⅔ cup creamy milk

1. Wash and drain the raspberries. Reserve 12 berries for decoration. Purée the rest of the fruit and pass through a sieve to remove the seeds.

2. Whisk together the water, syrup, egg yolks and cream. Pour into a double saucepan or into a basin standing over a pan of gently simmering water. Whisk until thickened, gradually beating in the milk. Cool.

3. Fold in the raspberry purée. Pour into a dish, cover and freeze for 2–3 hours, beating every 20 minutes to break down ice crystals.

4. Scoop into dessert dishes and decorate with the remaining raspberries.

about 380 kcal/1590 kJ

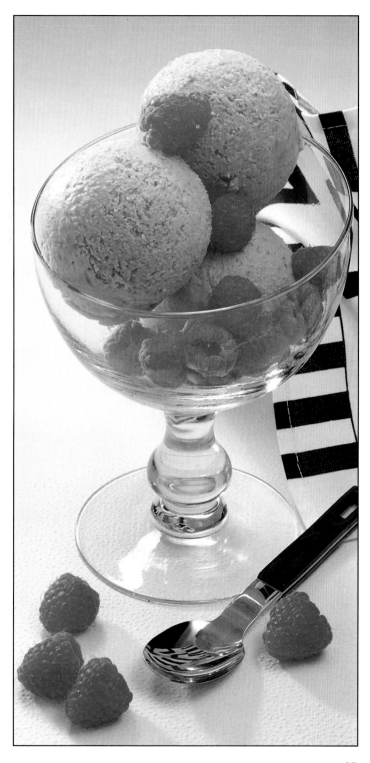

CHEESE CAKE ON A TRAY

Preparation time: 1¼ hours

Makes 20 pieces

For the dough:

150 g/5 oz/⅔ cup butter, melted

100 g/4 oz clear honey

250 g/9 oz quark, 20 per cent fat

10 ml/2 tsp finely grated lemon rind

1 egg yolk

sea salt

5 ml/1 tsp baking powder

350 g/12 oz/3 cups wholemeal flour

extra butter for greasing tray

For the filling:

75 g/3 oz raisins, soaked for 30 minutes in hot water

150 ml/¼ pt/⅔ cup whipping cream

375 ml/13 fl oz/1½ cups water

30 ml/2 tbsp cornflour

2 pinches of ground saffron

100 ml/3½ fl oz/6½ tbsp golden syrup, melted

750 g/1¾ lb quark, 20 per cent fat

finely grated rind of 1 large lemon

2 egg yolks

1. To make the dough, beat the melted butter to a smooth cream with the honey and quark. Add the lemon rind, egg yolk and a good pinch of sea salt. Mix thoroughly.

2. Combine the baking powder with the wholemeal flour and gradually fork into the quark mixture to make a firm dough.

3. Grease a large baking tray with butter. Cover with dough, pressing it out with back of a large damp tablespoon. Leave to stand for 15 minutes. Pre-heat the oven to 160°C/325°F/gas mark 3.

4. Meanwhile, prepare the filling. Drain the raisins thoroughly and pat dry with kitchen paper.

5. Mix the cream with the water. Remove 100 ml/3½ fl oz/½ cup and blend smoothly with the cornflour. Add the saffron and golden syrup. Pour into a large saucepan.

6. Whisk in the rest of the cream and water. Slowly bring to the boil, stirring all the time. Simmer gently for 2 minutes. Cool slightly.

7. Beat the cornflour mixture into the quark with the raisins, lemon rind and egg yolks. Reheat briefly until the mixture just comes up to the boil.

8. Spread smoothly over the dough. Bake for 35–40 minutes until the top is lightly browned. Cool on the tray and cut into portions when cold.

about 280 kcal/1170 kJ per piece

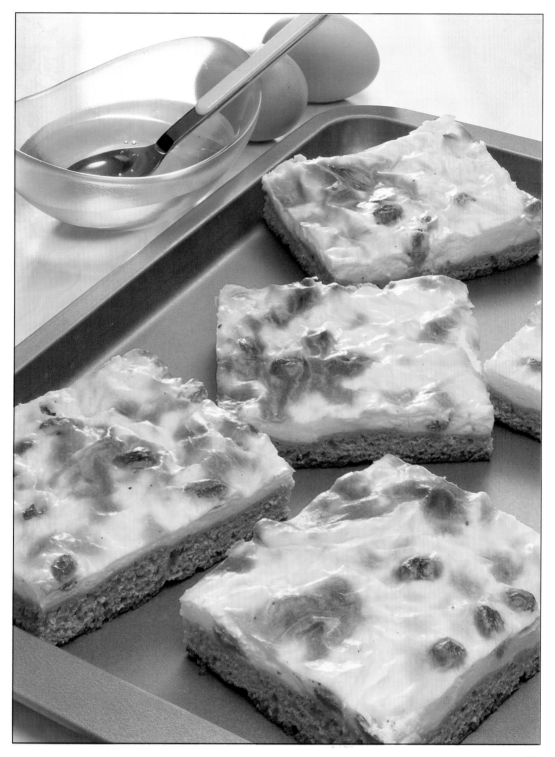

47

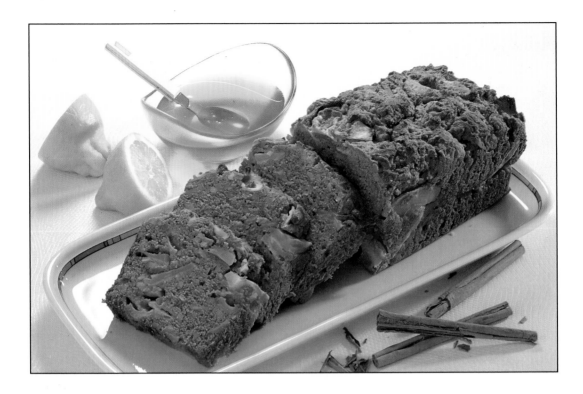

LOAF TIN CAKE WITH APPLE PIECES

Preparation time: 1¾ hours

Makes 15 pieces

100 g/4 oz/½ cup melted butter
100 g/4 oz clear honey
2 egg yolks
30 ml/2 tbsp whipping (heavy) cream
75 ml/5 tbsp water
finely grated rind of 1 medium lemon
100 g/4 oz coarsely chopped blanched almonds
2.5 ml/½ tsp sea salt
5 ml/1 tsp vanilla essence (extract)
7.5 ml/1½ tsp ground cinnamon
15 ml/1 tbsp baking powder
350 g/12 oz/3 cups wholemeal flour
350 g/12 oz eating apples, peeled, cored and sliced
extra butter for greasing baking tray

1. Mix the melted butter smoothly with the honey, egg yolks, cream and water. Add the lemon rind, almonds, salt, vanilla and cinnamon. Stir well to mix.

2. Combine the baking powder and wholemeal flour. Gradually add to the melted butter mixture, stirring until well blended. Stand for about 15 minutes. Preheat the oven to 160°C/325°F/gas mark 3.

3. Stir the prepared apples into the cake mixture. Grease a 1 kg/2 lb loaf tin with extra butter. Fill evenly with cake mixture then bake until well risen and golden. Turn out when lukewarm and cool completely on a wire rack.

about 270 kcal/1090 kJ per piece

Tips

To make the cake rise evenly, put a tin of cold water into the oven at the beginning of the baking.

Wrap the cold cake in foil to keep it moist.

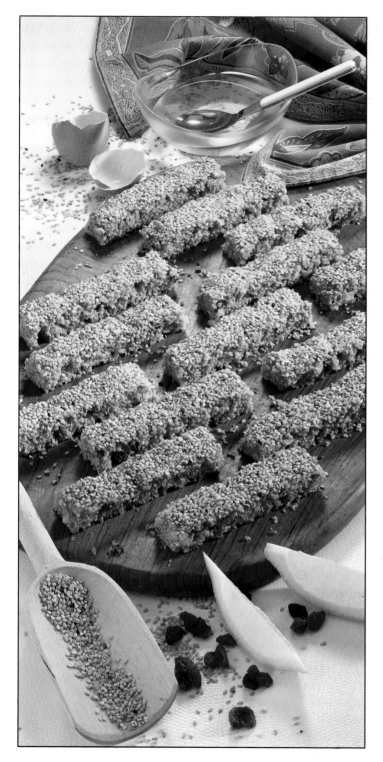

SESAME SLICES

Preparation time: 45 minutes

Makes 40 pieces

100 g/4 oz/½ cup melted butter
150 g/5 oz clear honey
250 ml/8 fl oz/1 cup buttermilk
finely grated rind of 1 medium lemon
1 egg yolk
100 g/4 oz chopped blanched almonds
100 g/4 oz raisins
2.5 ml/½ tsp sea salt
10 ml/2 tsp baking powder
350 g/12 oz/3 cups wholemeal flour
10 ml/2 tsp extra butter for greasing tray
milk for brushing
100 g/4 oz sesame seeds

1. Mix the melted butter with the honey and buttermilk until smooth. Add the lemon rind, egg yolk, almonds, raisins and salt. Stir until smooth.

2. Combine the baking powder with the flour and gradually stir into the buttermilk mixture. Preheat the oven to 160°C/ 325°F/gas mark 3.

3. Grease baking tray. Cover the base with the dough and leave to stand for 15 minutes. Finally, brush with milk and sprinkle with sesame seeds.

4. Bake for about 25 minutes until warm golden brown. Cool slightly then cut into about 40 narrow bars. Leave to cool on a wire rack.

about 120 kcal/500 kJ
per piece

FRENCH CARAWAY BISCUITS

Preparation time: 30 minutes

Cooling time: 30 minutes

Makes 40 pieces

200 g/7 oz/1¾ cups wholemeal flour
50 g/2 oz/¼ cup cold butter
100 g/4 oz quark, 20 per cent fat
2.5 ml/½ tsp sea salt
5 ml/1 tsp Provence herbs
5 ml/1 tsp margarine for greasing trays
1 egg yolk
15 ml/1 tbsp caraway seeds

1. Knead the flour to a pliable dough with the butter, quark, salt and herbs.

2. Working on a floured surface, shape the dough into a long sausage measuring about 3 cm/1¼ in in diameter. Wrap in foil. Refrigerate for 30 minutes.

3. Preheat the oven to 180°C/350°F/gas mark 4. Cut the roll into about 40 equal slices and place on greased baking trays.

4. Whisk the egg yolk with 2 tsp of water, brush the biscuits with this and sprinkle with caraway seeds. Bake for 15–18 minutes.

about 30 kcal/125 kJ per piece

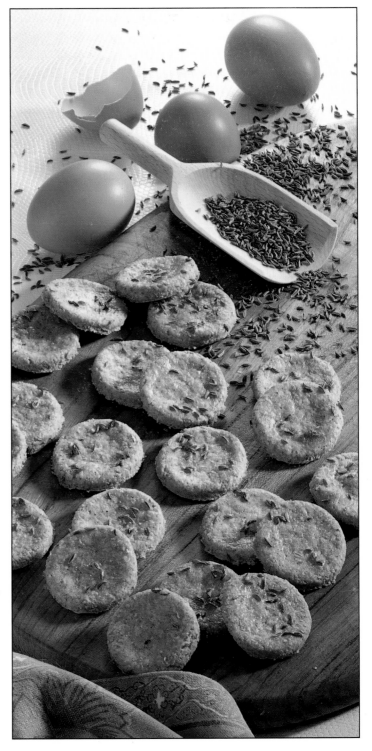

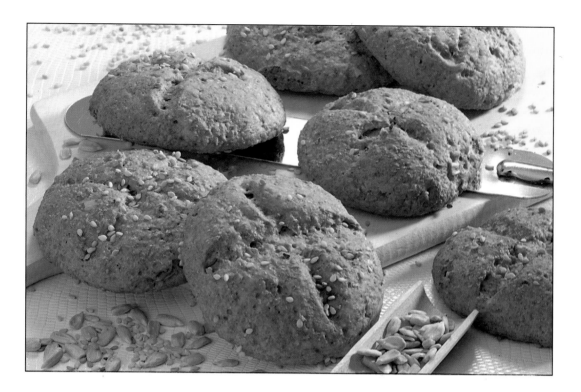

LITTLE GARLIC AND HERB BREAD ROLLS

Preparation time: 45 minutes
Rising time: 1 hour 20 minutes

Makes 30 rolls

1 sachet easy-blend dried yeast

200 ml/7 fl oz/scant 1 cup lukewarm water

½ kg/1 lb 1 oz wholemeal flour

120 ml/4 fl oz/½ cup buttermilk

2 medium onions, chopped

10 ml/2 tsp cold pressed sunflower or olive oil

1 clove garlic, finely chopped

2.5 ml/½ tsp coriander seeds, crushed

5 ml/1 tsp sea salt

5 ml/1 tsp dried oregano

5 ml/1 tsp dried thyme

50 g/2 oz sunflower seeds

margarine for greasing trays

1 egg yolk

20 ml/4 tsp sesame seeds

1. Tip the yeast, water, flour and buttermilk into a mixing bowl and work to a pliable dough. Knead on a floured surface until smooth and elastic. Cover and leave to rise in the warm for about 1 hour.

2. Fry the onions gently in the oil until transparent.

3. Knead the onions, garlic, coriander, salt, oregano, thyme and sunflower seeds into the risen dough. Grease 2 large baking trays with some margarine.

4. Preheat the oven to 200°C/400°F/gas mark 6. Shape the dough into 30 balls with floured hands. Arrange on the greased trays and cut a cross on top of each roll. Leave to rise in the warm for about 20 minutes or until doubled in size.

5. Brush the rolls with egg yolk and sprinkle with sesame seeds. Bake for 15–18 minutes. Cool on a wire rack.

about 105 kcal/440 kJ per roll

51

Small Salads and Starter Soups

RAW VEGETABLE SALAD

Preparation time: 20 minutes

Serves 2

For the salad:

3 carrots
1 small rettich (daikon)
100 g/4 oz mushrooms
1 small cucumber
1 red (bell) pepper
parsley for garnishing

For the dressing:

15 ml/1 tbsp sunflower oil
2.5 ml/½ tsp sea salt
10 ml/2 tsp lime juice
45 ml/3 tbsp water

1. Peel the carrots and the rettich. Wash and grate separately.

2. Clean the mushrooms, rinse quickly and slice thinly.

3. Peel the cucumber and slice very thinly.

4. Wash the pepper, de-seed and cut the flesh into strips or dice.

5. Place a little heap of grated carrot in the centre of each plate. Arrange the other raw vegetables individually around it.

6. Beat together dressing ingredients, pour over the raw vegetables and garnish with parsley.

about 130 kcal/545 kJ

Photograph opposite (top)

MUSHROOM SALAD

Preparation time: 35 minutes

Serves 2

For the salad:

400 g/14 oz green beans
sea salt
250 g/9 oz mushrooms
15 ml/1 tbsp butter
10 ml/2 tsp Italian seasoning
10 ml/2 tsp vegetarian vegetable stock (instant powder)
4 tomatoes
1 red (bell) pepper

For the dressing:

15 ml/1 tbsp cold pressed olive oil
15 ml/ 1 tbsp lemon juice
75 ml/5 tbsp water
5 ml/1 tsp herb salt

In addition:

10 ml/2 tsp chopped fresh parsley

1. Wash and string the beans then cut into 2.5 cm/1 in lengths. Cook until just soft in a little lightly salted water, allowing 15–18 minutes.

2. In the meantime, clean the mushrooms, wash quickly and slice thinly.

3. Melt the butter in a frying pan. Add the mushrooms and fry over a medium heat on all sides until they are lightly brown. Season with Italian seasoning and vegetable stock. Leave to cool.

4. Wash the tomatoes. Wash the pepper. Cut both into narrow strips.

5. Strain the beans and arrange on two plates. Add the mushrooms, tomatoes and pepper.

6. To make dressing, mix the olive oil and lemon juice with the water and season with herb salt.

7. Pour the dressing over the salad and garnish with parsley.

about 240 kcal/1000 kJ

Photograph opposite (centre)

KOHLRABI SALAD

Preparation time: 15 minutes

Serves 2

3 heads kohlrabi (about 550 g/1¼ lb)
150 ml/¼ pt/⅔ cup soured cream
50 ml/4 tbsp water
15 ml/1 tbsp lemon juice
5 ml/1 tsp herb salt
5 ml/1 tsp honey
30 ml/2 tbsp finely chopped fresh herbs (parsley, chives, dill)
15 ml/1 tbsp sunflower seeds

1. Peel the kohlrabi, wash and grate coarsely.

2. Stir the soured cream with the water, lemon juice, herb salt and honey.

3. When evenly combined, pour over the grated kohlrabi. Sprinkle the herbs and sunflower seeds over the top.

about 200 kcal/840 kJ

Photograph opposite (bottom)

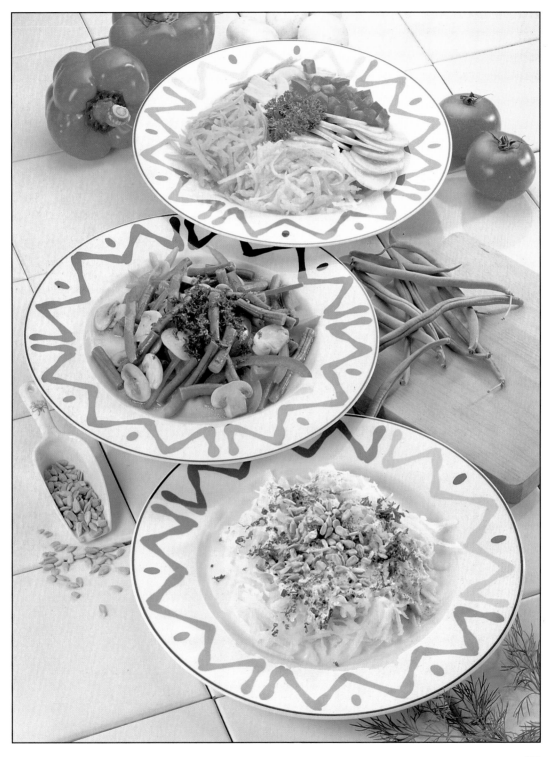

53

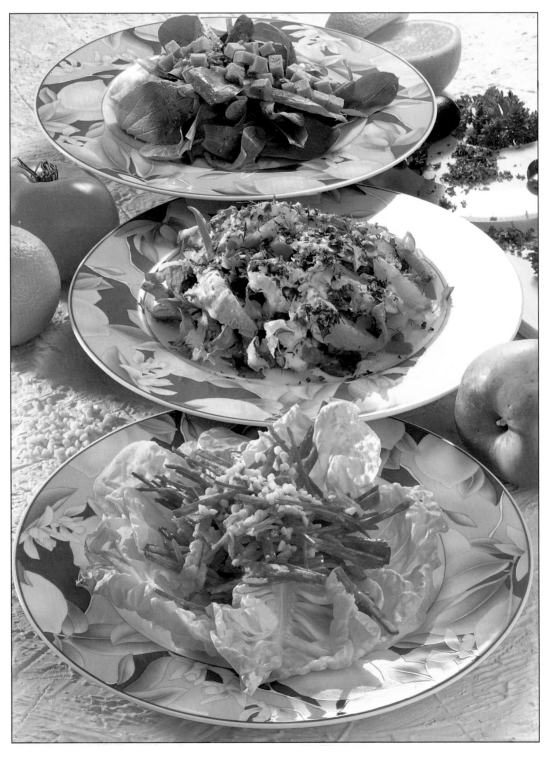

54

LAMBS' LETTUCE WITH CELERIAC AND TOFU

Preparation time: 1 hour

Serves 2

1 celeriac, about 400 g/14 oz
15 ml/1 tbsp lemon juice
100 g/4 oz lambs' lettuce or young spinach
50 g/2 oz smoked tofu
15 ml/1 tbsp sunflower oil
100 ml/3½ fl oz/6½ tbsp water
5 ml/1 tsp vegetarian vegetable stock (instant powder)
10 ml/2 tsp lemon juice
30 ml/2 tbsp chopped fresh chives

1. Wash the celeriac, cut it into chunks. Cook in plenty of water with the 1 tsp of lemon juice for 20–25 minutes. Leave to cool and grate coarsely. Divide between 2 plates.

2. Wash the lettuce or spinach, leave to drain and arrange on top of celeriac.

3. Dice the smoked tofu finely and fry in hot oil until golden brown. Remove and place on one side.

4. Pour the water into the frying pan, bring to the boil, season with vegetarian vegetable stock and add the lemon juice.

5. Leave the sauce to cool a little then pour over the salad while still warm. Top with tofu pieces then sprinkle with chopped chives.

about 125 kcal/520 kJ

Photograph opposite (top)

ENDIVE AND ORANGE SALAD

Preparation time: 30 minutes

Serves 2

For the salad:

1 small head of chicory
1 large red (bell) pepper
2 beef tomatoes
2 oranges

For the dressing:

2 oranges
150 ml/¼ pt/⅔ cup buttermilk or smetana
5 ml/1 tsp herb salt
5 ml/1 tsp honey
15 ml/1 tbsp chopped fresh herbs (chives, parsley, dill)

1. Wash and chop the chicory and put into a bowl.

2. Wash and halve the pepper, remove the inside fibres and seeds and cut the flesh into thin strips. Wash the tomatoes and also cut into strips. Add to the bowl.

3. Peel the oranges and remove the white pith. Cut out the segments in between the membranes with a sharp knife. Add to the bowl.

4. To make the dressing, squeeze the oranges and mix the juice with the buttermilk or smetana. Season with herb salt and honey.

5. Toss the dressing into salad then sprinkle with chopped herbs.

about 260 kcal/1090 kJ

Photograph opposite (centre)

BEETROOT AND APPLE SALAD

Preparation time: 20 minutes

Serves 2

1 green lettuce heart
400 g/14 oz uncooked beetroots
3 small Bramley apples
15 ml/1 tbsp lemon juice
30 ml/2 tbsp golden syrup or honey
150 ml/¼ pt/⅔ cup buttermilk or smetana
10 ml/2 tsp chopped blanched almonds

1. Clean the lettuce, remove any damaged leaves, wash and drain well. Arrange on 2 plates.

2. Wash the beetroots well, clean, peel and cut into fine sticks.

3. Wash the apples, quarter, remove the core and grate coarsely. Sprinkle with lemon juice.

4. Mix the beetroot with the apples and sweeten lightly with syrup or honey. Stir in the buttermilk or smetana.

5. Arrange the raw vegetables over the lettuce and sprinkle with almonds.

about 310 kcal/1300 kJ

Photograph opposite (bottom)

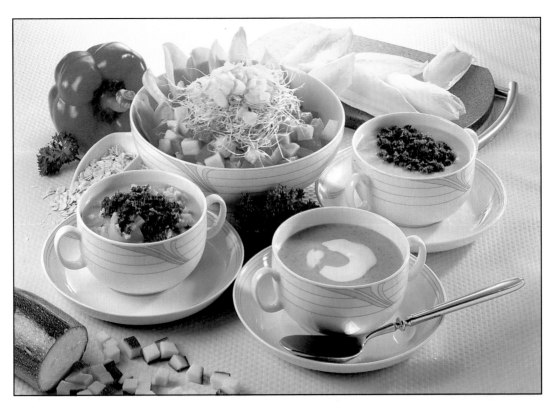

CHICORY SALAD WITH MANGO

Preparation time: 25 minutes

Serves 2

For the salad:

2 heads chicory	
2 red (bell) peppers	
1 large ripe mango	

For the dressing:

30 ml/2 tsp lemon juice	
75 ml/5 tbsp water	
10 ml/2 tsp honey	
15 ml/1 tbsp walnut oil	
5 ml/1 tsp sea salt	

For sprinkling on top:

50 g/2 oz alfalfa sprouts	
20 g/¾ oz flaked almonds	

1. Clean the chicory, wash, halve and cut out the bitter core at the base of each. Reserve 4 of the best leaves for garnishing. Finely chop the remaining leaves.

2. Wash the pepper, quarter and remove the seeds and white fibres. Cut the flesh into small dice.

3. Peel the mango, cut the flesh off the stone then dice.

4. Put the chicory into a bowl. Add the pepper and mango then garnish with the reserved chicory leaves.

5. To make the dressing, mix together the lemon juice, water, honey, oil and salt. Pour over the salad.

6. Rinse the alfalfa sprouts under cold running water and leave until well drained.

7. Before serving, sprinkle the alfalfa sprouts and the almonds over the salad.

about 270 kcal/1130 kJ

Photograph above (top)

Tip:

This salad goes very well with poultry or veal.

56

GRANDMA'S OAT SOUP

Preparation time: 30 minutes

Serves 2

1 large leek
300 g/11 oz carrots
200 g/7 oz celeriac
20 ml/4 tsp butter
100 g/4 oz coarse oatmeal
750 ml/1¼ pt/3 cups vegetarian vegetable stock (made from instant powder)
50 ml/2 fl oz/3½ tbsp single cream
30 ml/2 tbsp chopped fresh parsley

1. Slit and trim the leek, wash thoroughly and cut into fine rings. Peel the carrots and the celeriac, wash and dice finely.

2. Gently fry the vegetables in the butter until very pale gold.

3. Sprinkle with oatmeal and fry, stirring, for about 3 minutes.

4. Add the vegetable stock, a little at a time. Bring to the boil, stirring. Cover and simmer for 20 minutes over a low heat until the vegetables are tender. Stir frequently.

5. Stir in the cream and sprinkle with parsley.

about 410 kcal/1715 kJ

Photograph opposite (bottom left)

POTATO AND LEEK SOUP

Preparation time: 35 minutes

Serves 2

450 g/1 lb leeks
450 g/1 lb potatoes
15 ml/1 tbsp butter
750 ml/1¼ pt/3 cups hot water
15 ml/1 tbsp vegetarian vegetable stock (instant powder)
50 g/2 fl oz/3½ tbsp single cream
30 ml/2 tbsp chopped fresh parsley

1. Slit and trim the leeks, wash thoroughly and cut into 1 cm/ ½ in pieces. Wash the potatoes, peel and cut into small cubes.

2. Melt the butter in a saucepan. Add the leeks and potatoes and fry over a low heat until just beginning to colour.

3. Pour in the water and season the soup with vegetable stock powder. Bring to the boil, stirring. Cover and simmer for 15–18 minutes.

4. Purée the soup, return to the pan and bring just up to the boil. Stir in the cream and serve sprinkled with parsley.

about 320 kcal/1340 kJ

Photograph opposite (right)

COURGETTE SOUP

Preparation time: 40 minutes

Serves 2

800 g/1¾ lb courgettes (zucchini)
450 g/1 lb potatoes
1 clove garlic
1 onion
30 ml/2 tbsp butter
1 ltr/1¾ pt/4¼ cups hot water
15 ml/1 tsp vegetarian vegetable stock (instant powder)
50 ml/2 fl oz/3½ tbsp single cream

1. Wash and dry the courgettes then top and tail. Peel the potatoes and wash. Cut both vegetables into chunks.

2. Peel the garlic and onion. Chop finely and fry gently in a large saucepan with the butter until transparent. Add the courgettes and diced potato and continue to fry for about 5 minutes, stirring frequently.

3. Add the water then season with the vegetable stock. Cover and leave to simmer for 15–18 minutes, stirring two or three times.

4. Purée soup in a blender. Reheat before serving and stir in the cream.

about 350 kcal/1465 kJ

Photograph opposite (bottom centre)

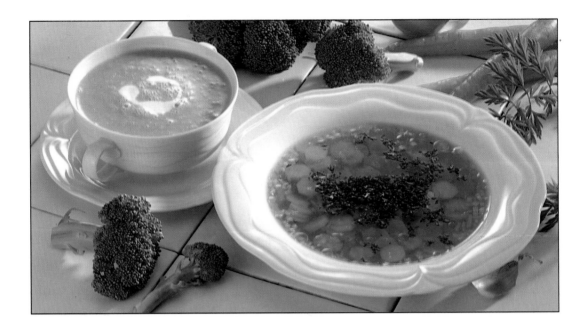

BROCCOLI CREAM SOUP

Preparation time: 25 minutes

Serves 2

450 g/1 lb broccoli

750 ml/1¼ pt/3 cups vegetarian vegetable stock (made from instant powder)

50 ml/2 fl oz/3½ tbsp single cream

1. Wash the broccoli thoroughly and divide into florets. Remove the stalks and slice thinly.

2. Put the florets and stalks into a saucepan. Add the vegetable stock, bring to boil, lower the heat and cover and simmer gently for 15–18 minutes.

3. Purée the soup in a food processor. Reheat until hot and stir in the cream.

about 115 kcal/480 kJ

Photograph above (left)

Variation

Other vegetables may be used instead of broccoli to include cauliflower, asparagus, carrots, leeks or peas.

Cream soups make a filling carbohydrate main meal when eaten with a wholemeal bread roll followed by a piece of cake as dessert.

CARROT SOUP

Preparation time: 35 minutes

Serves 2

1 small onion

250 g/9 oz carrots

15 ml/1 tbsp butter

500 ml/17 fl oz/2¼ cups vegetarian vegetable stock (made from instant powder)

15 ml/1 tbsp chopped fresh parsley

1. Peel the onion and chop finely. Wash, peel and slice thinly the carrots.

2. In a medium-sized saucepan, fry the onion in the butter until transparent. Add the carrot slices and fry for 7 minutes, turning frequently.

3. Pour in the vegetable stock and simmer, covered, for 15–20 minutes. Sprinkle each portion with parsley.

about 90 kcal/375 kJ

Photograph above (right)

Main Courses

'PEKING' SALAD

Soaking time: overnight
Preparation time: 35 minutes

Serves 2

For the salad:

100 g/4 oz brown rice

350 ml/13 fl oz/1½ cups water

200 g/7 oz young spinach leaves

4 spring onions

150 g/5 oz mushrooms

8 cherry tomatoes

For the dressing:

20 ml/4 tsp sunflower oil

5 ml/1 tsp herb salt

10 ml/2 tsp lemon juice

75 ml/5 tbsp water

In addition:

150 g/5 oz fresh bean sprouts

1. Cover the rice with water and leave to soak overnight.

2. Next day, cook the rice in its soaking water over a low heat for about 25 minutes. Drain and rinse.

3. Wash the spinach and tear into small pieces. Wash the spring onions and cut into very fine rings. Clean the mushrooms, wash briefly and slice thinly. Wash and halve the tomatoes.

4. Mix the prepared salad ingredients in a large bowl with the rice.

5. To make the dressing, stir together the oil, herb salt, lemon juice and water. Toss into the salad, then sprinkle with washed sprouts.

about 330 kcal/1380 kJ

Variation

Instead of spinach leaves you can also use fine slivers of carrots, peas or diced (bell) pepper.

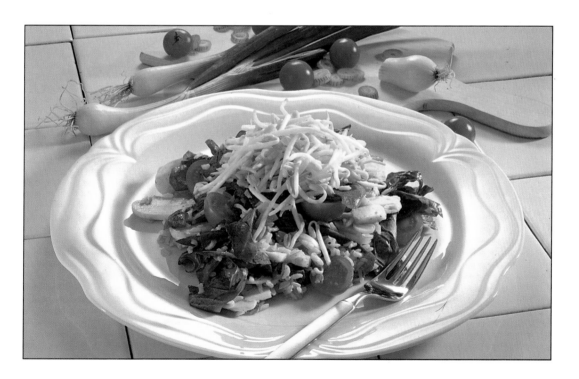

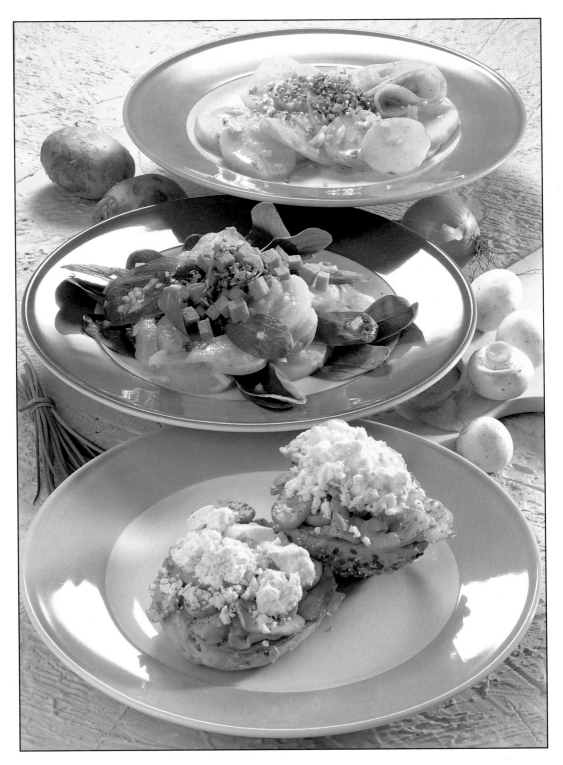

POTATO AND CELERIAC SALAD

Preparation time: 50 minutes

Serves 2

1 celeriac about 400 g/14 oz
450 g/1 lb potatoes, boiled in skins
100 ml/3½ fl oz/6½ tsp buttermilk or smetana
10 ml/2 tsp sunflower oil
10 ml/2 tsp lemon juice
30 ml/2 tbsp water
5 ml/1 tsp herb salt
5 ml/1 tsp honey
1 onion, chopped
15 ml/1 tbsp chopped fresh chives

1. Wash the celeriac well and cook in plenty of salted water for 20–25 minutes or until tender. When cold, peel and slice thinly.

2. Peel the boiled potatoes and slice. Mix with the celeriac in a large bowl.

3. To make the dressing, stir together the buttermilk or smetana, oil, water, lemon juice, herb salt and honey. Add the onion.

4. Pour the dressing over the salad, toss well and sprinkle with the chives.

about 315 kcal/1320 kJ

Photograph opposite (top)

SAVOURY POTATO SALAD

Preparation time: 30 minutes

Serves 2

450 g/1 lb potatoes, boiled in skins
100 g/4 oz lambs' lettuce or baby spinach
1 onion
50 g/2 oz smoked tofu, diced
10 ml/2 tsp sunflower oil
175 ml/6 fl oz/¾ cup vegetarian vegetable stock
10 ml/2 tsp lemon juice
15 ml/1 tbsp chopped fresh chives

1. Peel the boiled potatoes and slice into a large bowl.

2. Wash the lambs' lettuce or spinach well and then drain.

3. Peel the onion, chop finely and add to the potatoes with the lettuce or spinach.

4. Fry the tofu in hot oil until golden brown. Drain on kitchen paper.

5. Add the vegetable stock to the frying pan, heat to lukewarm then pour on to the salad with the lemon juice.

6. Sprinkle with tofu and chives.

about 210 kcal/880 kJ

Photograph opposite (centre)

CHEESEY TOASTED BREAD ROLL

Preparation time: 20 minutes

Serves 2

2 onions
8 mushrooms
10 ml/2 tsp butter
5 ml/1 tsp herb salt
2 wholemeal bread rolls
100 g/4 oz sheeps' cheese, crumbled

1. Peel the onions and chop finely. Clean the mushrooms, wash quickly and slice thinly.

2. Heat the butter in a frying pan. Add onions and mushrooms and fry fairly briskly until all the liquid has evaporated. Season with herb salt.

3. Halve the rolls and toast until golden brown.

4. Top with onion and mushroom mixture then sprinkle with crumbled cheese.

about 340 kcal/1420 kJ

Photograph opposite (bottom)

Tip

Eat a neutral salad with this (see page 52).

OYSTER MUSHROOM SOUP

Preparation time: 35 minutes

Serves 2

450 g/1 lb floury potatoes
400 g/14 oz oyster mushrooms
1 onion
15 ml/1 tbsp butter
750 ml/1¼ pt/3 cups water
15 ml/1 tbsp vegetarian vegetable stock powder
2 cloves garlic
10 ml/2 tsp chopped fresh parsley

1. Wash the potatoes, peel and dice.

2. Clean the oyster mushrooms, rinse quickly and cut into narrow strips.

3. Peel the onion, chop finely and fry gently until transparent in the butter. Add the potatoes and mushrooms and stir-fry for 3 minutes.

4. Add the water and vegetable stock. Crush in the garlic, cover and cook the soup over a low heat for 15–18 minutes.

5. Stir round and serve each portion sprinkled with parsley.

about 270 kcal/1130 kJ

Photograph opposite (top left)

CARROT AND POTATO SOUP

Preparation time: 30 minutes

Serves 2

600 g/1 lb 6 oz carrots
450 g/1 lb potatoes
1 onion
10 ml/2 tsp butter
750 ml/1¼ pt/3 cups vegetarian vegetable stock
30 ml/2 tbsp cream
5 ml/1 tsp chopped fresh parsley

1. Wash the carrots and potatoes. Peel thinly and cut into chunks. Peel the onion and chop.

2. Melt the butter in a saucepan. Add the carrots, potatoes and onion. Pour in the stock. Bring the soup to the boil, cover then simmer for 15–18 minutes.

3. Purée the soup in a food processor. Reheat, stir in the cream and serve sprinkled with parsley.

about 350 kcal/1460 kJ

Photograph opposite (top right)

WHOLEMEAL BAGUETTE WITH PIQUANT SAUERKRAUT SALAD

Preparation time: 20 minutes

Serves 2

½ red (bell) pepper
1 tomato
1 small onion
150 g/5 oz sauerkraut
1 clove garlic
5 ml/1 tsp preserved green peppercorns
5 ml/1 tsp sunflower oil
5 ml/1 tsp honey
2 wholemeal bread rolls, crisply baked

1. Rinse the pepper, remove the seeds and cut the flesh into strips. Wash the tomato. Peel the onion and chop finely.

2. Mix the prepared vegetables with the sauerkraut.

3. Crush in the garlic then add the peppercorns and sunflower oil. Mix everything well and sweeten with honey.

4. Halve the rolls and toast. Place plenty of sauerkraut salad on top of each. Should any salad remain, eat with the bread rolls.

about 480 kcal/2010 kJ

Photograph opposite (below)

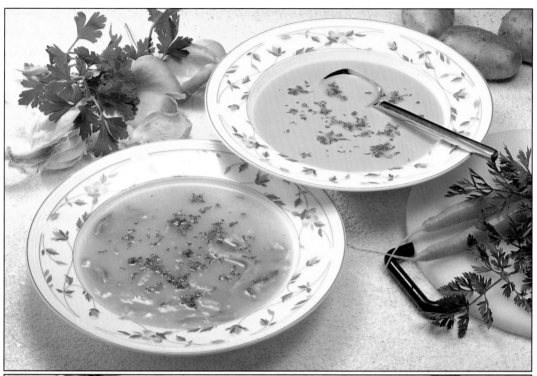

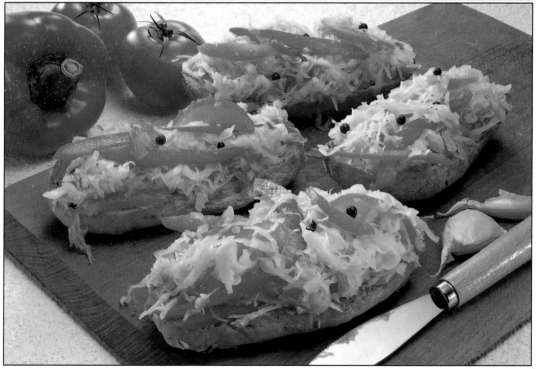

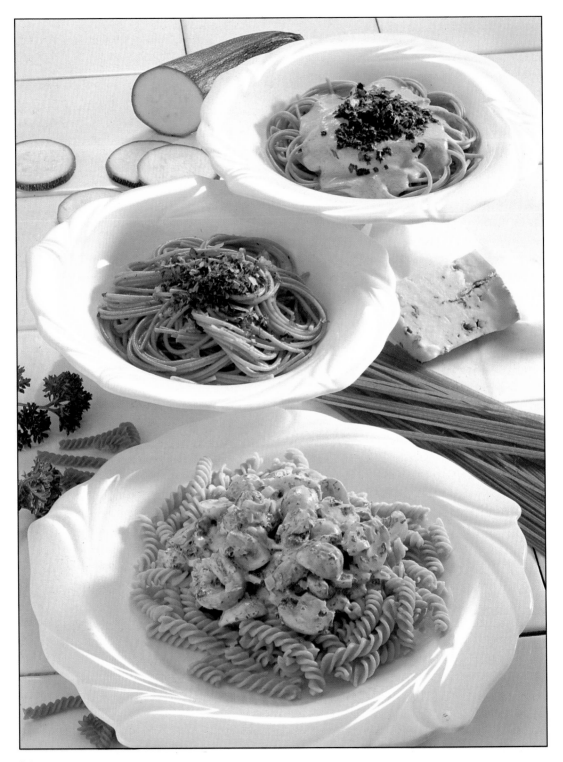

SPAGHETTI WITH COURGETTE SAUCE

Preparation time: 20 minutes

Serves 2

150 g/5 oz wholemeal spaghetti
sea salt
600 g/1¼ lb courgettes
15 ml/1 tbsp butter
1 clove garlic
10 ml/2 tsp vegetarian vegetable stock (instant powder)
75 g/3 oz Gorgonzola or similar blue cheese with 60 per cent fat
30 ml/2 tbsp soured (dairy sour) cream
30 ml/2 tbsp chopped fresh basil

1. Cook the spaghetti in plenty of boiling salted water for about 10 minutes until *al dente*.

2. Meanwhile, wash the courgettes, top and tail then slice very thinly.

3. Melt the butter in a frying pan, add the courgettes and fry gently for 5 minutes. Crush in the garlic then season with the vegetarian vegetable stock. Cover and simmer for about 10 minutes, stirring twice.

4. Cut the cheese into small dice, add to the pan and allow to melt.

5. Just before serving, stir in the soured cream. Purée in a food processor. Reheat gently until hot.

6. Drain the spaghetti, arrange on plates then coat with the sauce. Garnish by sprinkling with basil.

about 550 kcal/2300 kJ

Photograph opposite (top)

SPAGHETTI WITH GARLIC SAUCE

Preparation time: 20 minutes

Serves 2

150 g/5 oz wholemeal spaghetti
1 clove garlic
sea salt
30 ml/2 tbsp olive oil
2.5 ml/½ tsp herb salt
a pinch of cayenne pepper
15 ml/1 tbsp chopped fresh marjoram

1. Cook the spaghetti in plenty of lightly salted boiling water until *al dente*; about 10 minutes.

2. Meanwhile, peel the garlic and crush into a saucepan. Add the oil. Season with herb salt and cayenne pepper.

3. Drain the spaghetti and toss with the garlic oil. Serve on warm plates, sprinkle with the marjoram.

about 420 kcal/1760 kJ

Photograph opposite (centre)

Tip

A neutral tomato salad or sliced tomatoes go well with the pasta.

NOODLES WITH MUSHROOM CREAM SAUCE

Preparation time: 45 minutes

Serves 2

350 g/12 oz mushrooms
1 onion
15 ml/1 tbsp butter
300 ml/½ pt/1¼ cups vegetarian vegetable stock
60 ml/4 tbsp cream
15 ml/1 tbsp chopped fresh parsley
100 g/4 oz wholemeal twist-shaped pasta
sea salt

1. Clean and wash the mushrooms and chop finely. Peel the onion and finely chop.

2. Melt the butter in a frying pan. Add the onion and fry gently until transparent. Add the mushrooms and fry over a medium heat for 3 minutes.

3. Pour stock over the mushrooms, cover the pan and simmer for 20–25 minutes, stirring twice.

4. Meanwhile, cook the pasta in lightly salted boiling water for about 10 minutes until *al dente*. Drain. Arrange on warm plates.

5. Stir the cream and parsley into the mushroom mixture. Adjust salt to taste and spoon over noodles.

about 400 kcal/1675 kJ

Photograph opposite (bottom)

Tip

Eat this with a neutral salad (see page 52)

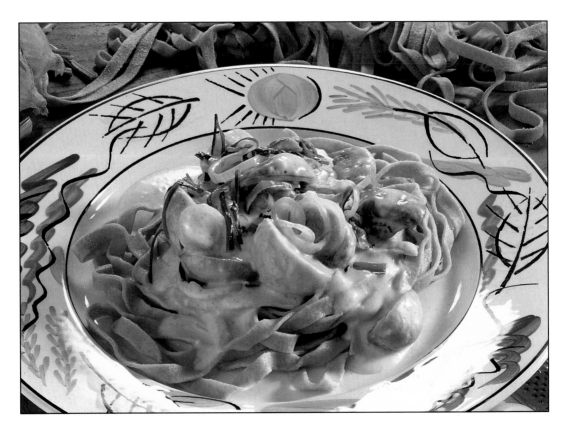

TAGLIATELLE WITH VEGETABLE AND CHEESE SAUCE

Preparation time: 40 minutes

Serves 2

1 leek
1 onion
150 g/5 oz small mushrooms
15 ml/1 tbsp butter
20 ml/4 tsp wholemeal flour
300 ml/½ pt/1¼ cups water
45 ml/3 tbsp single cream
10 ml/2 tsp vegetarian vegetable stock (instant powder)
grated nutmeg
100 g/4 oz wholemeal tagliatelli
sea salt
75 g/3 oz Cheddar cheese, chopped

1. Halve the leek lengthwise, wash thoroughly and cut into narrow strips. Peel the onion and slice thinly.

2. Separate the onions into rings. Clean the mushrooms, wash quickly and halve.

3. Melt the butter in a frying pan. Add the leek, onions and mushrooms and fry for 15 minutes over medium heat. Sprinkle with wholemeal flour. Fry for 30 seconds, stirring.

4. Add the water and cream. Season with vegetable stock and nutmeg. Cover and simmer gently for 10 minutes.

5. In the meantime, cook the noodles in lightly salted boiling water for about 10 minutes until *al dente*. Drain.

6. Add the cheese to the vegetable and mushroom sauce and heat gently until melted, stirring all the time.

7. Serve the noodles topped with the sauce.

about 590 kcal/2470 kJ

Tip

Eat with a neutral salad (see page 52).

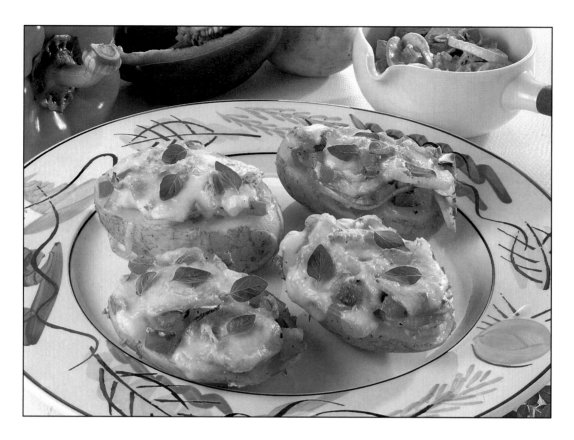

FILLED OVEN POTATOES

Preparation time: 1 hour

Serves 2

4 potatoes, each 150 g/5 oz
1 large onion
200 g/7 oz mushrooms
2 red (bell) peppers
1 green (bell) pepper
10 ml/2 tsp butter
10 ml/2 tsp vegetarian vegetable stock (instant powder)
5 ml/1 tsp crushed dried oregano
5 ml/1 tsp butter for the baking dish
100 g/4 oz Mozzarella cheese
15 ml/1 tbsp soured (dairy sour) cream
few small mint leaves for garnishing

1. Wash the potatoes and cook for 12 minutes in a saucepan with just enough water to cover. Drain and leave to cool completely.

2. Peel onion, thinly slice and separate into rings. Wash the mushrooms briefly and slice. Wash the peppers, halve, remove the inside fibres and seeds and fairly finely chop.

3. Fry the onion rings, mushrooms and peppers gently in the butter in a pan. Season with vegetarian stock and oregano. Preheat the oven to 200°C/400°F/gas mark 6.

4. Halve the potatoes along the length and remove the centres with a teaspoon. Place the halves in a buttered heatproof dish and place some of the vegetables in the hollows.

5. Dice the cheese and sprinkle over the filling. Bake the potatoes in the oven for about 15 minutes.

6. Mix the rest of the vegetables with the soured cream and serve as an accompaniment to the potatoes. Garnish with mint leaves.

about 580 kcal/2345 kJ

BOILED POTATOES WITH TSATZIKI

Preparation time: 30 minutes

Serves 2

450 g/1 lb potatoes
250 g/9 oz quark, 20 per cent fat
45 ml/3 tbsp mineral water
2 cloves garlic
1 medium cucumber
herb salt
1 sprig of dill

1. Brush the potatoes clean under cold running water. Boil in their skins for 18–20 minutes. Drain.

2. Meanwhile, prepare the tsatziki. Mix the quark with the mineral water, then peel and crush in the garlic.

3. Peel 150 g/5 oz of the cucumber and grate. Add to the quark and season with herb salt.

4. Peel the remainder of the cucumber and slice. Serve the boiled potatoes with the tsatziki and cucumber slices. Garnish with the dill.

about 300 kcal/1255 kJ

Photograph opposite (top)

PAN PIZZA

Time to rise: about 1 hour 20 minutes

Preparation time: 1 hour 15 minutes

Serves 6

For the dough:

1 sachet easy-blend dried yeast
300 ml/½ pt lukewarm water
450 g/1 lb wholemeal flour
5 ml/1 tsp sea salt
10 ml/2 tsp olive oil
butter for greasing tray

For the filling:

3 red (bell) peppers
200 g/7 oz mushrooms
1 onion
10 ml/2 tsp olive oil
10 ml/2 tsp vegetarian vegetable stock (instant powder)
10 ml/2 tsp crushed dried oregano
100 g/4 oz stoned green olives
200 g/7 oz Mozzarella cheese
1 sprig of marjoram, chopped

1. Tip the yeast, water, flour, salt and olive oil into a large bowl and work to a pliable dough. Knead on a floured surface until smooth and elastic. Cover and leave to rise in the warm for about 1 hour.

2. Grease a large baking tray (Swiss roll tin) with butter. Spread the dough evenly over the base. Prick with a fork all over so that no bubbles form during baking. Cover the dough again and leave in a warm place for about 20 minutes to rise. Preheat the oven to 200°C/400°F/gas mark 6.

3. Meanwhile, wash the peppers then halve and de-seed. Rinse and drain the mushrooms. Cut both into thin strips.

4. Fry the vegetables briefly in a pan in the olive oil. Season with vegetarian vegetable stock and oregano.

5. Spread the vegetables and the olives over the dough. Dice the cheese and sprinkle over the top, followed by the marjoram.

6. Bake the pizza for about 25 minutes until the cheese has melted and the crust is crisp and golden brown.

about 360 kcal/1510 kJ

Photograph opposite (below)

Tip

Eat with a neutral salad (see page 52).

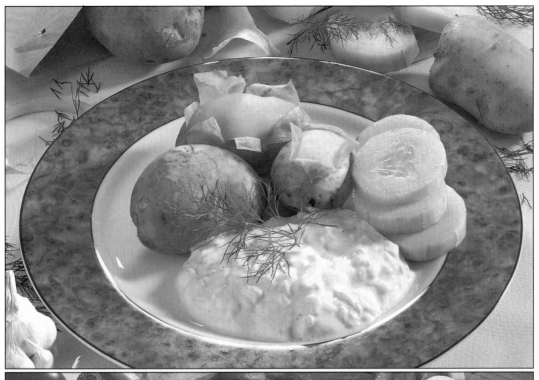

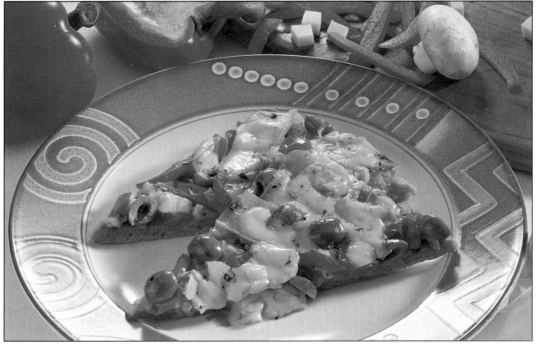

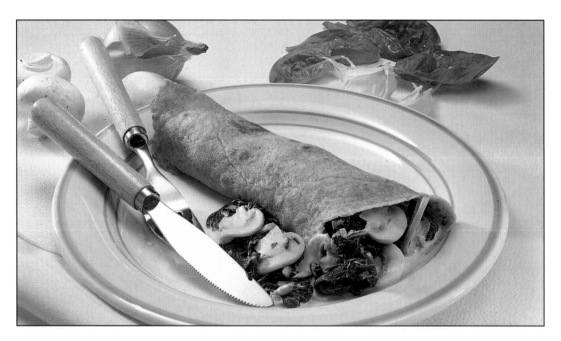

PIQUANT FILLED PANCAKES

Preparation time: 45 minutes

Serves 2

For the pancakes:

100 ml/3½ fl oz/6½ tsp single cream
300 ml/½ pt/1¼ cups water
2.5 ml/½ tsp sea salt
2 egg yolks
150 g/5 oz/1¼ cups wholemeal flour
1 tsp baking powder
2 tbsp sunflower oil

For the filling:

450 g/1 lb spinach
1 medium onion
150 g/5 oz mushrooms
5 ml/1 tsp butter
20 ml/4 tbsp sunflower seeds
10 ml/2 tsp vegetarian vegetable stock (instant powder)
1 clove garlic
20 ml/4 tsp soured (dairy sour) cream
1 large pinch of grated nutmeg

1. To make the batter, whisk the cream, water, salt and egg yolks in a large bowl.

2. Gradually beat in the wholemeal flour sifted with baking powder. When smooth and creamy looking, cover and refrigerate while preparing the rest of the ingredients.

3. Wash the spinach for the filling and quickly blanch in boiling water. Drain.

4. Peel the onion and finely chop. Wash the mushrooms briefly and cut into thin slices.

5. Melt the butter in a frying pan, add the onion and fry gently until transparent. Add the mushrooms with the sunflower seeds and fry for about 10 minutes over a low heat, stirring frequently.

6. Chop the spinach coarsely and add to the onion and mushroom mixture. Season with vegetable stock then crush in the peeled garlic.

7. Thicken the mixture by adding the soured cream. Season with nutmeg.

8. Heat the oil in a non-stick frying pan and fry 4 small or 2 large pancakes from the batter.

9. Spread some of the vegetables on each and roll up. Serve with the remaining vegetables.

about 950 kcal/4000 kJ

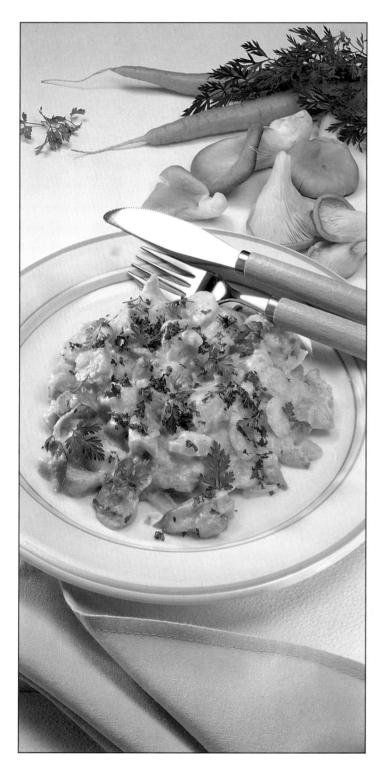

OYSTER MUSHROOM RAGOUT

Preparation time: 30 minutes

Serves 2

400 g/14 oz carrots
400 g/14 oz oyster mushrooms
1 onion
15 ml/1 tbsp butter
30 ml/2 tbsp wholemeal flour
300 ml/½ pt/1¼ cups vegetarian vegetable stock
30 ml/2 tbsp soured (dairy sour) cream
20 ml/4 tsp chopped fresh parsley
20 ml/4 tsp fresh chervil leaves

1. Peel and wash the carrots then cut into thin slices.

2. Clean the oyster mushrooms, wash quickly and chop coarsely.

3. Peel the onion and finely chop. Melt the butter in a frying pan, add the onion and fry until transparent. Add the carrots and mushrooms. Continue to stir-fry for 5 minutes.

4. Sprinkle with flour, pour on vegetable stock and stir well. Bring to the boil, lower the heat and cover. Simmer gently for 15–20 minutes.

5. Mix in the soured cream and sprinkle each portion with the parsley and chervil.

about 250 kcal/1050 kJ

Tip

As this belongs to the carbohydrate group, you can eat it with mashed potato (see page 92) or rice.

MUSHROOM AND MILLET RISSOTTO

Preparation time: 35 minutes

Serves 2

250 g/9 oz mushrooms
1 onion
10 ml/2 tsp butter
100 g/4 oz frozen peas
10 ml/2 tsp curry powder
100 g/4 oz millet
1 clove garlic
10 ml/2 tsp vegetarian vegetable stock (instant powder)
450 ml/¾ pt/2 cups hot water
45 ml/3 tbsp single (light) cream
15 ml/1 tbsp finely chopped fresh parsley

1. Rinse the mushrooms, drain and cut into fine slices. Peel the onion and finely chop.

2. Melt the butter in a frying pan. Add the mushrooms and onion and fry for 3–4 minutes, stirring. Add the peas and sprinkle with curry powder.

3. Rinse the millet with hot water and add to the vegetables. Crush in the garlic then season with vegetable stock.

4. Pour in the water, bring to the boil, lower the heat and cover. Simmer the rissotto for 20–25 minutes when the millet should be soft. Stir several times.

5. Fork in the cream and sprinkle each portion with parsley.

about 405 kcal/1690 kJ

Tip

Accompany with a fresh neutral salad or a neutral raw vegetable platter (see page 52).

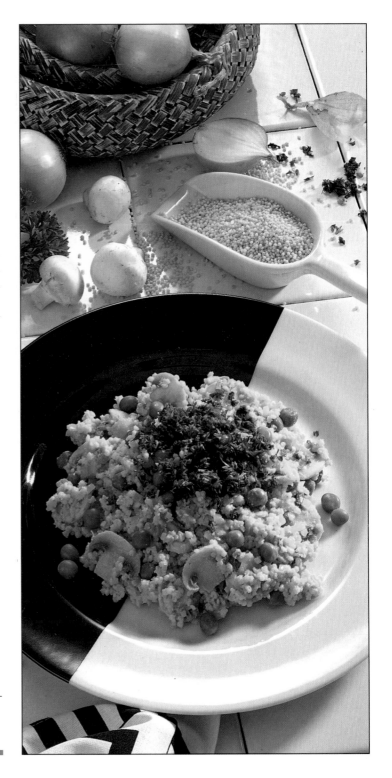

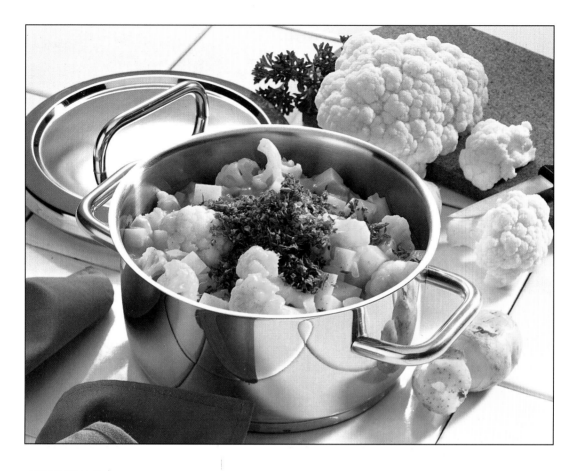

CURRY POT

Preparation time: 30 minutes

Serves 2

1 large cauliflower
450 g/1 lb potatoes
5 ml/1 tsp sea salt
1 onion
30 ml/2 tbsp butter
30 ml/2 tbsp curry powder
45 ml/3 tbsp wholemeal flour
30 ml/2 tbsp cream
10 ml/2 tsp vegetarian vegetable stock (instant powder)
20 ml/4 tsp chopped fresh parsley

1. Trim the cauliflower, wash and break into tiny florets. Wash the potatoes, peel and dice. Cook both together in 900 ml/ 1½ pt/3¾ cups of lightly salted water. Drain, reserving the cooking liquor.

2. Peel the onion, chop and fry in the butter in a large pan until transparent. Sprinkle with the curry and flour and cook for ½ minute, stirring. Add 300 ml/ ½ pt/1¼ cups of cooking liquor little by little, stirring all the time.

3. Slowly bring to the boil, stirring continually and simmer for about 5 minutes until it thickens. If necessary, add extra water as it should not be too thick. Stir in the cream and season with the vegetable stock powder.

4. Add the cauliflower and the potatoes, reheat until hot and sprinkle each portion with parsley.

about 540 kcal/2260 kJ

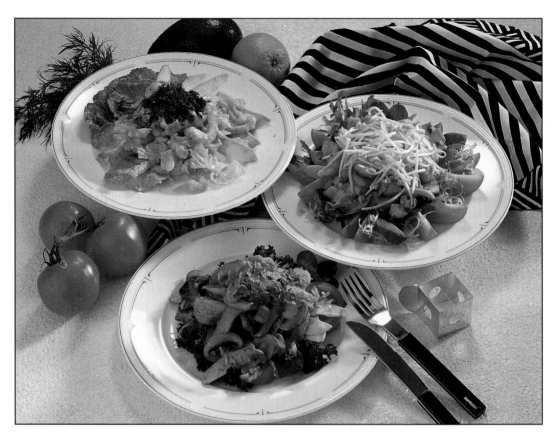

PRAWN SALAD

Preparation time: 25 minutes

Serves 2

For the salad:

1 crisp lettuce
2 oranges
1 avocado
200 g/7 oz peeled prawns, thawed if frozen

For the dressing:

75 ml/5 tbsp freshly squeezed orange juice
1 large pinch of cayenne pepper
5 ml/1 tsp honey
5 ml/1 tsp sea salt
120 ml/4 fl oz/½ cup soured (dairy sour) cream
30 ml/2 tbsp chopped fresh dill

1. Wash and drain the lettuce then tear large leaves into bite-size pieces. Arrange the smaller leaves in a fan-shaped pattern on flat plates.

2. Peel the oranges and remove the pith. Cut the flesh into small pieces, discarding the pips.

3. Peel the avocado, halve and stone. Cut the flesh into narrow segments. Arrange the rest of the lettuce leaves with the oranges and the avocado, on the plates. Pat prawns dry with kitchen paper.

4. To make the dressing, stir the orange juice with the cayenne pepper, honey and salt then whisk in soured cream.

5. Pour the dressing over the salad. Top with the prawns then sprinkle with chopped dill.

about 450 kcal/1880 kJ

Photograph above (left)

74

HEALTHY SALAD

Preparation time: 1 hour

Serves 2

For the salad:

275 g/10 oz chicken breast fillet
100 g/4 oz mushrooms
20 ml/4 tsp sunflower oil
sea salt to taste
1 small frisée lettuce
100 g/4 oz lambs' lettuce or young spinach
3 tomatoes
½ fresh pineapple
2 large carrots

For the dressing:

150 g/¼ pt/⅔ cup buttermilk or smetana
5 ml/1 tsp honey
10 ml/2 tsp lemon juice
5 ml/1 tsp herb salt

For sprinkling:

100 g/4 oz mung or soy bean sprouts

1. Wash the chicken, pat dry with kitchen paper and cut into small pieces. Wash the mushrooms and slice thinly.

2. Heat the oil in a frying pan. Add the chicken and mushrooms and fry for about 10 minutes, stirring. Season with salt and leave to cool.

3. Wash the salad leaves, drain thoroughly and tear into bite-size pieces. Wash the tomatoes. Cut each into eighths. Arrange the leaves and tomatoes on plates.

4. Peel the pineapple, quarter along the length and cut out the hard stalk. Cut the flesh into small pieces. Peel the carrots and grate coarsely.

5. To make the dressing, lightly whisk the buttermilk or smetana with the honey, lemon juice and herb salt.

6. Mix the pineapple and the carrots with the dressing and spoon over the salad.

7. Arrange the chicken and mushrooms on top. Sprinkle with sprouts.

about 440 kcal/1840 kJ

Photograph above (right)

TURKEY AND AVOCADO SALAD

Preparation time: 45 minutes

Serves 2

For the salad:

2 portions of turkey breast fillet, each 150 g/5 oz
8 mushrooms
10 ml/2 tsp margarine
5 ml/1 tsp herb salt
1 small oak leaf lettuce
1 small lollo rosso lettuce
3 tomatoes
1 ripe avocado

For the dressing:

1 small onion
10 ml/2 tsp sunflower oil
5 ml/1 tsp herb salt
15ml/1 tbsp lemon juice
75 ml/5 tbsp water
15 ml/1 tbsp chervil leaves

1. Wash the turkey, pat dry with kitchen paper and cut into small strips. Clean the mushrooms, wash quickly and cut into very thin slices.

2. Heat the margarine in a frying pan. Add the turkey and mushrooms and fry briskly for 3 minutes. Season with herb salt. Half-cover and simmer for another 8 minutes. Stir from time to time. Leave on one side.

3. Wash and drain the lettuce then tear the leaves into bite-size pieces. Wash the tomatoes and cut each into eighths.

4. Halve the avocado down the length and remove the stone. Peel the avocado halves and cut the flesh into thin segments.

5. To make the dressing, peel the onion and chop finely. Beat together the oil, herb salt, lemon juice and water. Add the onion.

6. Arrange the lettuce leaves, tomatoes and avocado segments on plates. Sprinkle with the dressing then top with warm turkey and mushrooms. Garnish with chervil leaves.

about 490 kcal/2050 kJ

Photograph opposite (bottom)

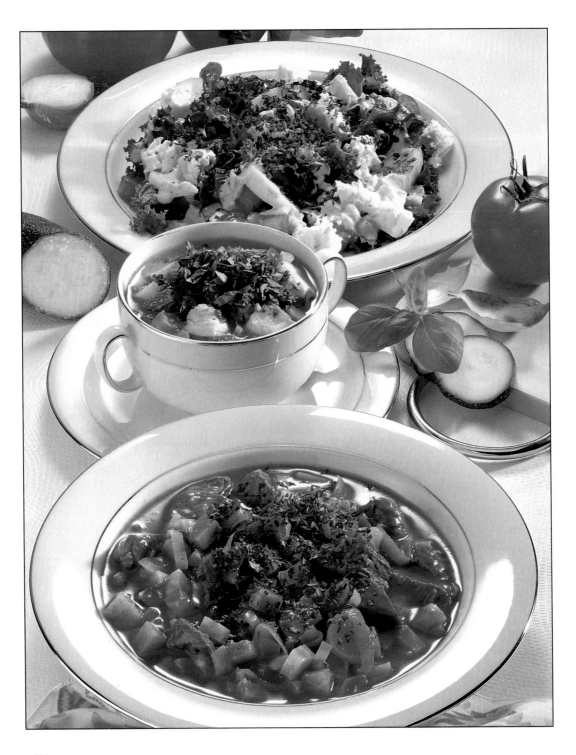

MIXED FARM SALAD

Preparation time: 20 minutes

Serves 2

1 small lollo rosso lettuce
1 small oak leaf lettuce
2 beef tomatoes
2 eating apples
100 g/4 oz mild sheeps' cheese
10 ml/2 tsp lemon juice
45 ml/3 tbsp water
2.5 ml/½ tsp herb salt
20 ml/1½ tbsp soured (dairy sour) cream
5 ml/1 tsp honey
1 onion
20 ml/4 tsp finely chopped herbs (parsley, chervil, cress)

1. Wash and drain both lettuces and tear the leaves into bite-sized pieces.

2. Wash and dry the tomatoes and cut the flesh into small pieces.

3. Peel the apples, quarter, remove the core and cut the flesh into thin slices.

4. Mix the lettuce, tomatoes and apples in a bowl. Add the cheese in pieces.

5. To make the dressing, whisk together the lemon juice, water and soured cream. Season with herb salt and honey.

6. Peel the onion, chop finely and add to the dressing.

7. Toss the salad with the dressing and sprinkle with the chopped herbs.

about 290 kcal/1210 kJ

Photograph opposite (top)

SPANISH CHICKEN SOUP

Preparation time: 45 minutes

Serves 2

2 celery stalks
1 onion
4 sprigs of parsley
1 clove garlic, crushed
10 ml/2 tsp cold pressed olive oil
350 g/12 oz chicken breast fillet
750 ml/1¼ pt/2 cups water
1 red (bell) pepper
1 courgette (zucchini)
3 tomatoes
15 ml/1 tbsp vegetarian vegetable stock (instant powder)
5 ml/1 tsp crushed dried oregano
5 ml/1 tsp crushed dried rosemary
15 ml/1 tbsp chopped fresh basil

1. Wash the celery and thinly slice. Put into a large saucepan.
2. Peel the onion and chop finely. Add to the pan with the celery, parsley, crushed garlic and olive oil. Fry gently for 5 minutes, stirring twice.
3. Wash the chicken, pat dry and cut into walnut-sized pieces. Add to the vegetables. Top up with water.
4. Wash the pepper, cut in half and remove the inside fibres and seeds. Top and tail the the courgette then wash and dry. Cut both into small dice.
5. Blanch the tomatoes, remove the skins and chop coarsely. Add to the pan with the pepper and courgette. Season with vegetable stock, oregano and rosemary. Bring to the boil, lower the heat and cover.
6. Simmer for 20–25 minutes. Sprinkle with basil leaves.
about 320 kcal/1340 kJ

Photograph opposite (centre)

VEGETABLE POT WITH BEEF

Preparation time: 1½ hours

Serves 2

350 g/12 oz lean braising steak
20 ml/1½ tbsp margarine
10 ml/2 tsp paprika
1 large pinch of cayenne pepper
1 bay leaf
5 ml/1 tsp caraway seeds
5 ml/1 tsp herb salt
450 ml/¾ pt/2 cups vegetarian vegetable stock
2 leeks
1 onion
350 g/12 oz carrots
200 g/7 oz celeriac
15 ml/1 tbsp chopped fresh parsley

1. Rinse the meat, pat dry with kitchen paper and cut into small cubes.

2. Heat the margarine in a saucepan, add the meat and fry briskly until well browned. Add the paprika, cayenne pepper, bay leaf, caraway seeds and herb salt.

3. Pour in the vegetable stock, bring to the boil, lower the heat and cover. Simmer for 1–1¼ hours or until the meat is tender.

4. Slit the leek, wash well and cut into rings. Peel the onion, carrots and celeriac and cut into small dice.

5. When the meat is just cooked, add the vegetables and cover. Simmer for a further 20 minutes.

6. Before serving, remove the bay leaf and sprinkle each portion with parsley.

about 480 kcal/2010 kJ

Photograph opposite (bottom)

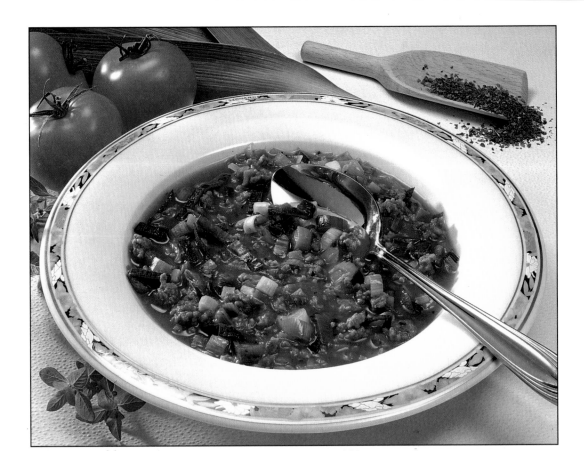

LEEK POT WITH MINCED MEAT AND TOMATO

Preparation time: 35 minutes

Serves 2

3 medium leeks
5 ml/1 tsp butter
350 g/12 oz minced steak
450 g/1 lb tomatoes
90 ml/6 tbsp water
10 ml/2 tsp vegetarian vegetable stock (instant powder)
5 ml/1 tsp crushed dried rosemary
5 ml/1 tsp crushed dried oregano
20 ml/1½ tbsp single (light) cream

1. Trim the leeks, halve lengthwise then wsah thoroughly and cut into thin rings.

2. Melt the butter in a saucepan, add the meat and stir-fry until brown and crumbly. Add the leek and fry for 5 minutes. Stir once or twice.

3. Blanch and skin the tomatoes, cut into quarters and work to purée in blender. Add to the meat.

4. Add the water then season with vegetable stock, rosemary and oregano and stir in the cream. Bring to the boil, lower the heat and cover. Simmer for 20 minutes, stirring twice.

about 585 kcal/2450 kJ

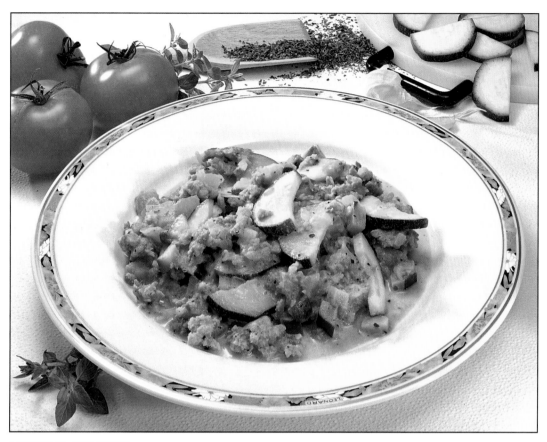

ITALIAN MINCED MEAT FRY

Preparation time: 45 minutes

Serves 2

1 aubergine
sea salt
2 courgettes (zucchini)
5 tomatoes
1 onion
1 clove garlic
15 ml/1 tbsp olive oil
350 g/12 oz minced steak
6 tbsp water
5 ml/1 tsp crushed dried rosemary
5 ml/1 tsp crushed dried oregano
5 ml/1 tsp vegetarian vegetable stock (instant powder)
30 ml/2 tbsp single (light) cream

1. Wash and dry the aubergine and cut into small cubes. Sprinkle with salt and leave to stand for 20 minutes. Pat dry with kitchen paper.

2. Wash the courgette and halve lengthwise. Blanch and skin the tomatoes then chop coarsely.

3. Peel the onion and garlic and chop both finely.

4. Heat the oil in a saucepan. Add the minced steak with the onion and garlic. Stir-fry until the meat is dry and crumbly.

5. Add the aubergine and courgette and fry for 5 minutes. Mix in the tomatoes and water. Bring to the boil, lower the heat and cover. Simmer for 20 minutes, stirring twice.

6. Stir in all the remaining ingredients and reheat briefly.

about 560 kcal/2340 kJ

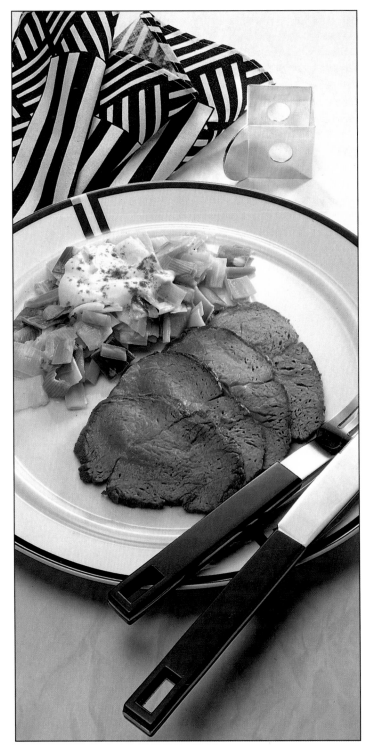

FILLET OF BEEF WITH LEEK

Preparation time: 35 minutes

Serves 2

3 large leeks
15 ml/1 tbsp butter
150 ml/¼ pt/⅔ cup vegetarian vegetable stock
45 ml/3 tbsp single (light) cream
350 g/12 oz beef fillet
10 ml/2 tsp sea salt
15 ml/1 tbsp margarine
20 ml/1½ tbsp soured (dairy sour) cream
5 ml/1 tsp paprika

1. Trim the leeks, halve each lengthwise and wash thoroughly. Cut into 1 cm/½ in slices.

2. Melt the butter in a saucepan. Add the leek and fry gently until soft, stirring frequently. Mix in the vegetable stock, bring to the boil, lower the heat and cover. Simmer for about 10 minutes. Stir in the cream.

3. Rinse the beef, pat dry with kitchen paper and rub in the salt. Heat the margarine in a frying pan, add the beef and fry until well browned on all sides. Cover. Simmer over a gentle heat for 20 minutes.

4. Cut the meat into slices and arrange on plates with the leeks. Top the leeks with cream and sprinkle with paprika.

about 560 kcal/2340 kJ

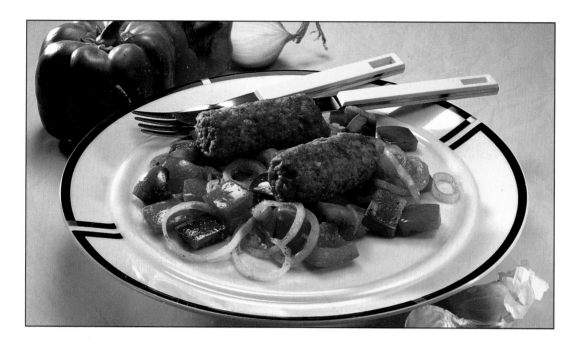

SPICED SAUSAGES AND PEPPERS

Preparation time: 45 minutes

Serves 2

For the vegetables:

1 medium-sized onion
2 red (bell) peppers
2 green (bell) peppers
10 ml/2 tsp sunflower oil
10 ml/2 tsp vegetarian vegetable stock (instant powder)
5 ml/1 tsp paprika

For the sausages:

1 small onion
1 egg, beaten
300 g/10 oz minced (ground) steak
5 ml/1 tsp sea salt
1 large pinch of cayenne pepper
10 ml/2 tsp olive oil

1. Peel and slice the onions then separate slices into rings. Wash the peppers and wipe dry. Halve, remove the inside fibres and seeds then cut the flesh into 2.5 cm/1 in cubes.

2. Heat the oil in a non-stick frying pan. Add the onion and pepper and stir-fry for 10 minutes.

3. Season the vegetables with the vegetable stock and paprika. Add water as necessary. Cover and cook over a low heat until *al dente*.

4. Meanwhile, peel the onion for the sausages and chop finely. Peel and crush the garlic. Add the onion, garlic and egg to the minced steak with salt and cayenne pepper.

5. Mix until smoothly combined using your hands or a fork.

6. Divide into 2 equal portions and shape into croquettes.

7. Heat the oil in a frying pan. Add the croquettes and fry on all sides until crispy brown. Reduce the heat and fry a total of 10 minutes, turning 2 or 3 times.

8. Place the vegetables on warmed plates and top with the sausages.

about 540 kcal/2270 kJ

Tip:

The vegetables above can also be served with the beef fillet recipe (see page 80) instead of leeks.

BEEFSTEAK ON MIXED VEGETABLES

Preparation time: 30 minutes

Serves 2

2 courgettes (zucchini)
1 large red (bell) pepper
1 large yellow (bell) pepper
4 carrots
15 ml/1 tbsp butter
75 ml/5 tbsp water
10 ml/2 tsp vegetarian vegetable stock (instant powder)
350 g/12 oz top quality minced (ground) steak or minced (ground) rump steak
5 ml/1 tsp sea salt
10 ml/2 tsp sunflower oil
1 onion
30 ml/2 tbsp chopped fresh parsley

1. Wash and dry the courgettes. Wash, halve and de-seed the peppers. Clean and peel the carrots. Cut the vegetables into strips.

2. Melt the butter in a frying pan, add the vegetables and fry gently for 7 minutes. Stir twice. Add the water, cover and cook for 5–10 minutes over a low heat until *al dente*. Season with vegetable stock.

3. Knead the minced meat with the salt and form into 4 burgers. Fry in the hot oil on both sides for 6 minutes, turning twice.

4. Peel the onion, cut into thin rings and fry with the burgers for 3 minutes.

5. Arrange the vegetables on plates with burgers and onions. Sprinkle with parsley to garnish.

about 430 kcal/1800 kJ

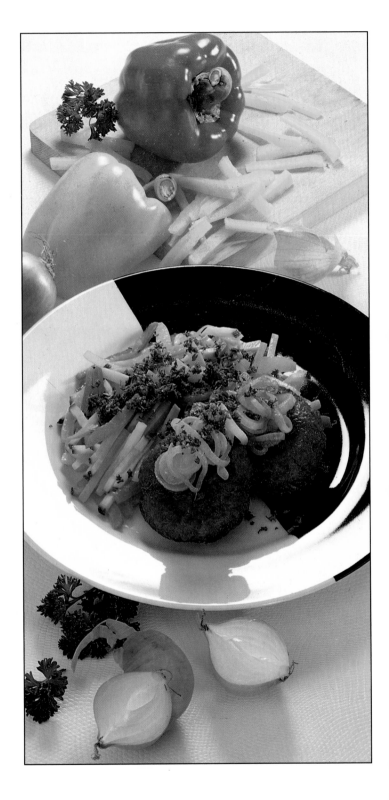

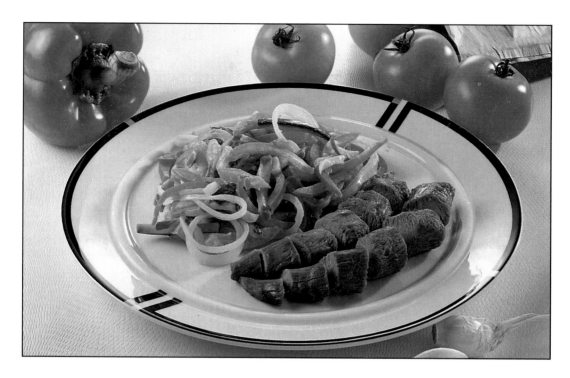

RATATOUILLE WITH LAMB FILLET

Preparation time: 40 minutes

Serves 2

For the ratatouille:

1 large onion
1 small aubergine
2 red (bell) peppers
1 courgette (zucchini)
2 tsp olive oil
1 clove garlic
4 tomatoes
5 ml/1 tsp Italian herb seasoning
10 ml/2 tsp vegetarian vegetable stock (instant powder)
30 ml/2 tbsp single cream

For the lamb fillets:

350 ml/12 oz lamb fillet (2 pieces)
sea salt
15 ml/3 tsp olive oil

1. Peel the onion and cut into thin slices then separate slices into rings. Wash and dry the aubergines, peppers and courgette. Cut all three into narrow strips, first de-seeding the peppers.

2. Heat the oil in a frying pan. Add the onions and fry until transparent. Crush in the peeled garlic. Add the rest of the vegetables and fry over a moderate heat for 5–8 minutes.

3. Blanch and skin the tomatoes then chop very finely.

4. Add the vegetables. Season with Italian herbs and stock. Cover. Simmer a further 10–15 minutes. Stir in the cream.

5. Wash the lamb fillets, pat dry and salt lightly. Heat the oil in a frying pan. Add the lamb and fry on each side for 4 minutes.

6. Serve with the ratatouille vegetables.

about 610 kcal/2550 kJ

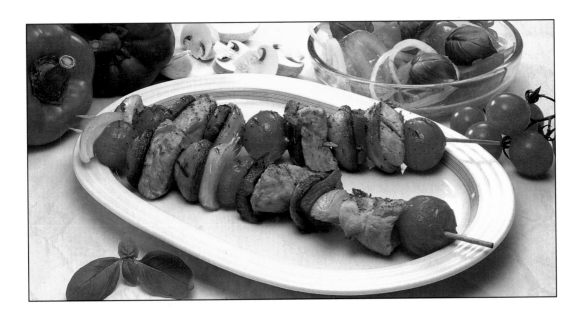

TURKEY KEBAB WITH TOMATO SALAD

Preparation time: 55 minutes

Serves 2

For the salad:

450 g/1 lb beef tomatoes
1 onion
5 ml/1 tsp herb salt
5 ml/1 tsp sunflower oil
1 sprig of basil

For the kebabs:

1 red (bell) pepper
1 green (bell) pepper
4 onions
12 cherry tomatoes
12 small mushrooms
300 g/12 oz turkey breast fillet
30 ml/2 tbsp lemon juice
45 ml/3 tbsp sunflower oil
5 ml/1 tsp chopped fresh thyme
5 ml/1 tsp salt
5 ml/1 tsp paprika
1 clove garlic

1. To make the salad, wash and dry the tomatoes, then cut into small squares. Put into a bowl.

2. Peel and slice the onions. Separate the slices into rings and add to the tomatoes.

3. Season with herb salt, sprinkle with sunflower oil and garnish with basil leaves. Leave on one side for the time being.

4. To make the kebabs, wash and dry the peppers then halve and de-seed. Cut the flesh into 2.5 cm/1 in squares.

5. Peel the onions and quarter. Wash the tomatoes and dry thoroughly.

6. Clean mushrooms, wash quickly and twist out the stalks.

7. Rinse the turkey, pat dry with kitchen paper and cut into 2 cm/¾ in cubes.

8. Arrange turkey and vegetables alternately onto skewers and sprinkle with lemon juice.

9. Make the marinade by beating together the sunflower oil, thyme, salt and paprika then add the peeled and crushed garlic.

10. Brush the kebabs all over with the marinade. Grill for 20–25 minutes turning frequently and brushing with remaining marinade.

about 510 kcal/2140 kJ

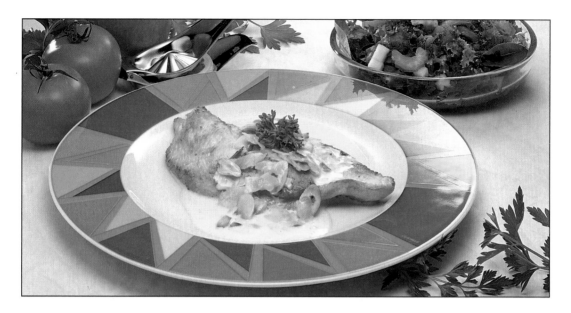

TURKEY SLICES WITH SUMMER SALAD

Preparation time: 35 minutes

Serves 2

For the salad:

1 large apple
15 ml/1 tbsp lemon juice
4 celery sticks
1 small lollo rosso lettuce
75 g/3 oz lambs' lettuce or young spinach
3 tomatoes

For the dressing:

10 ml/2 tsp sunflower oil
15 ml/1 tbsp lemon juice
100 ml/3½ fl oz/6½ tbsp water
5 ml/1 tsp herb salt
5 ml/1 tsp honey
15 ml/1 tbsp chopped fresh parsley

For the turkey slices:

2 turkey breast fillets, each 150 g/5 oz
5 ml/1 tsp herb salt
15 ml/1 tsp margarine
20 ml/4 tsp flaked almonds
75 ml/5 tbsp single cream
45 ml/3 tbsp water

1. Wash the apple, quarter and remove the core. Cut the flesh into small pieces and sprinkle with lemon juice.

2. Wash the celery then slice thinly. Wash the lettuce and lambs' lettuce or spinach. Pat dry with kitchen paper and tear into bite-sized pieces.

3. Wash the tomatoes, wipe dry and cut into small cubes. Put into a large bowl. Add the lettuce.

4. To make dressing, beat the oil with the lemon juice and water. Season with herb salt, honey and chopped parsley.

5. Pour over the salad and toss well to mix.

6. Wash the turkey, wipe dry with kitchen paper and season with herb salt.

7. In a frying pan, fry the turkey slices on both sides in margarine for 4–5 minutes, turning twice. Remove to warm plate.

8. Add the flaked almonds to the pan and fry for 1 minute, turning all the time. Replace the turkey. Add the cream and water then season with extra herb salt.

9. Serve the turkey coated with sauce. Accompany with salad.

about 500 kcal/2090 kJ

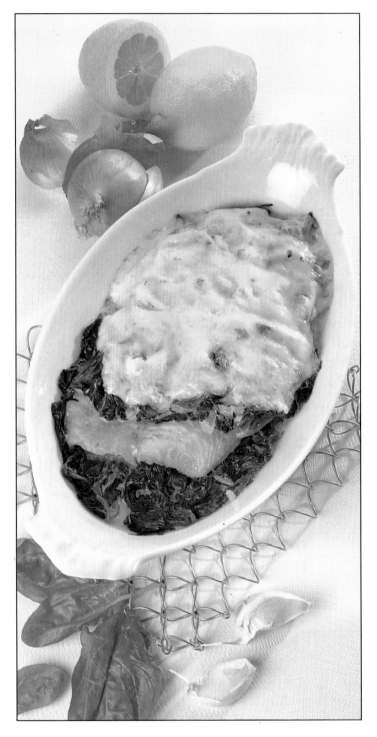

FISH GRATIN

Preparation time: 1¼ hours

Serves 2

600 g/1¼ lb spinach leaves
1 onion
10 ml/2 tsp sunflower oil
10 ml/2 tsp vegetarian vegetable stock (instant powder)
30 ml/2 tbsp single cream
1 clove garlic
400 g/14 oz salmon trout or salmon fillets, skinned
20 ml/4 tsp lemon juice
5 ml/1 tsp sea salt
100 g/4 oz Emmental cheese

1. Wash the spinach well, then blanch quickly in boiling water. Drain well and cut into coarse shreds. Reserve the blanching water.

2. Peel the onion and chop finely. Heat the oil in a frying pan, add the onions and fry gently until transparent. Add the spinach. Season with vegetable stock. Add the cream and 75 ml/3 fl oz/5 tbsp of the blanching water. Crush in the peeled garlic.

3. Preheat the oven to 200°C/400°F/gas mark 6. Sprinkle the fish fillets with the lemon juice and salt lightly.

4. Place half the spinach mixture in a soufflé dish and place the fish fillets on top. Cover with the rest of the spinach.

5. Cut the cheese into thin slices and place over the spinach. Bake for 20–25 minutes until golden brown.

about 530 kcal/2220 kJ

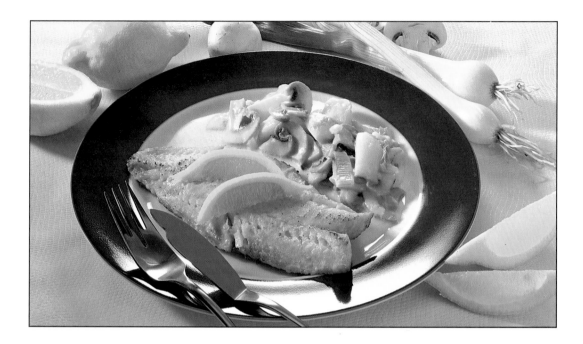

FISH FILLET WITH MUSHROOM SAUCE

Preparation time: 45 minutes

Serves 2

For the sauce:

1 bunch spring onions
400 g/14 oz mushrooms
10 ml/2 tsp butter
10 ml/2 tsp lemon juice
300 ml/½ pt/1¼ cups vegetarian vegetable stock
1 large pinch of saffron powder
50 ml/2 fl oz/3½ tbsp single cream
20 ml/1½ tbsp cornflour

For the fish:

400 g/14 oz white fish fillets (haddock, plaice, cod, coley or sole)
5 ml/1 tsp sea salt
20 ml/4 tsp sunflower oil
4 lemon wedges

1. Trim the spring onions, wash well then chop coarsely. Wipe the mushrooms, rinse and cut into thin slices.

2 Melt the butter in a frying pan. Add the onion and the mushrooms and fry for 5 minutes. Sprinkle with lemon juice. Add the vegetable stock.

3. Mix the saffron and cream together then combine smoothly with the cornflour. Pour into the pan over the onions and mushrooms. Bring to the boil, stirring. Leave over minimal heat.

4. In a second frying pan (non-stick for preference) fry the fish fillets in the oil for 5–7 minutes depending on thickness. Turn once.

5. Put on to warm plates, serve the sauce on the side and garnish with lemon wedges.

about 490 kcal/2050 kJ

Tip:

Eat this with a neutral salad (see page 52).

SCRAMBLED EGGS WITH MUSHROOMS

Preparation time: 20 minutes

Serves 2

200 g/14 oz mushrooms
1 onion
10 ml/2 tsp sunflower oil
4 eggs
75 ml/3 fl oz/6½ tbsp mineral water
230 ml/2 tbsp single (light) cream
sea salt
15 ml/1 tbsp chopped fresh chives

1. Wipe the mushrooms, rinse and cut into thin slices. Peel the onion and chop finely.

2. Heat the oil in a frying pan, add the mushrooms and onion and fry for 5 minutes, stirring.

3. Whisk the eggs with the mineral water and cream. Season to taste with salt. Stir in the chives.

4. Pour the egg mixture in the frying pan over the mushrooms and stir until scrambled over a low heat.

about 345 kcal/1440 kJ

Photograph opposite (top)

Tip

Eat a fresh neutral or protein salad with the scrambled eggs (see pages 52–56).

BROCCOLI EGG GRATIN

Preparation time: 50 minutes

Serves 2

450 g/1 lb broccoli
sea salt
1 onion
10 ml/2 tsp sunflower oil
4 tomatoes
4 eggs
100 ml/3½ fl oz/6½ tbsp soured (dairy sour) cream
10 ml/2 tsp vegetarian vegetable stock (instant powder)
5 ml/1 tsp butter for greasing dish
40 g/1½ oz Parmesan cheese, grated

1. Clean the broccoli and wash then divide into small florets. Cut off the stalks, then peel and cut into 2 cm/¾ in pieces. Cook the broccoli and stalks in boiling water for 10 minutes until *al dente*.

2. Peel the onion and slice. Fry quickly in a pan in the oil. Leave aside for the time being.

3. Blanch the tomatoes, remove the skins and cut in quarters. Purée in blender. Preheat oven to 180°C/350°F/gas mark 4.

4. Beat the eggs then whisk in the tomato purée, soured cream and vegetable stock.

5. Grease a gratin dish with butter and cover the base with broccoli and onion. Pour on the egg mixture, sprinkle with Parmesan cheese and bake for about 20 minutes until golden and crusty.

about 525 kcal/2200 kJ

Photograph opposite (centre)

LITTLE PLAICE ROLLS

Preparation time: 30 minutes

Serves 2

2 oranges
400 g/14 oz plaice fillets
5 ml/1 tsp herb salt
10 ml/2 tsp butter
100 ml/3½ fl oz/6½ tbsp water
30 ml/2 tbsp single cream
30 ml/2 tbsp chopped fresh dill

1. Squeeze out the juice of 1 orange. Peel the second orange, removing the white pith. Using a sharp knife, cut out segments of orange, leaving behind the coarse membrane 'dividers'.

2. Wash the plaice fillets, dry, cut lengthways into strips of 2.5 cm/1 in and salt lightly.

3. Place 1 orange segment on each strip of fish, roll up then hold in place with a cocktail stick.

4. Melt the butter in a frying pan, add the plaice rolls and fry briskly for 2 minutes, turning. Pour on the water and orange juice. Cover the fish and simmer for 8 minutes over a low heat.

5. Gently stir in the cream. Reheat without boiling. Sprinkle each serving with dill.

about 320 kcal/1340 kJ

Photograph opposite (bottom)

Tip

Eat with a neutral or a protein salad (see pages 52–56).

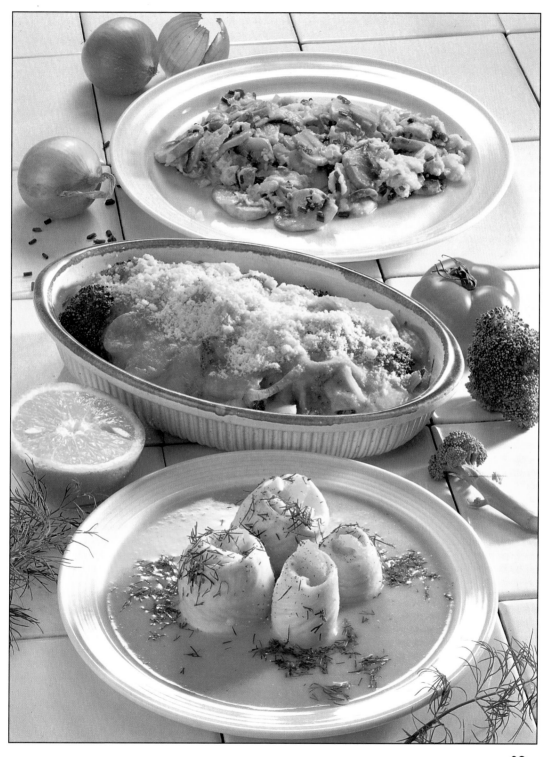

89

Vegetables, Accompaniments and Sauces ▬▬▬▬

MARROW MIX

Preparation time: 25 minutes

Serves 2

1 small marrow of about 800 g/1¾ lb
1 onion
15 ml/1 tsp butter
15 ml/1 tbsp curry powder
150 ml/¼ pt/⅔ cup vegetarian vegetable stock
50 ml/2 fl oz/3½ tbsp single (light) cream
20 ml/4 tsp chopped fresh dill

1. Peel the marrow, halve lengthwise and remove the seeds. Cut each half into thinnish slices.

2. Peel the onion, chop finely and fry in the butter in a large pan until transparent. Add the marrow and fry for 5 minutes.

3. Sprinkle with curry powder, pour on the vegetable stock and bring to the boil. Lower the heat, cover and cook for about 10–15 minutes until the marrow is tender.

4. Stir in the cream and spoon into a dish. Sprinkle with dill.

about 180 kcal/750 kJ

Photograph opposite (top)

Tip

This dish belongs to the neutral group. Should you wish to eat a protein meal, serve it with meat, fish or eggs. Should you prefer a carbohydrate meal, serve with rice, potatoes, pasta or cereals.

HONEY CARROTS

Preparation time: 25 minutes

Serves 2

800 g/1¾ lb carrots
15 ml/1 tbsp butter
200 ml/7 fl oz/scant 1 cup vegetable stock (instant powder)
10 ml/2 tsp vegetarian vegetable stock (instant powder)
5 ml/1 tsp honey
15 ml/1 tbsp chopped fresh parsley

1. Peel the carrots and cut into small cubes.

2. Melt the butter in a saucepan, add the carrots and stir-fry for 6 minutes. Add the stock and bring to the boil. Lower the heat and cover. Simmer for 15–20 minutes until tender.

3. Season with vegetable stock and honey. Serve sprinkled with parsley.

about 170 kcal/710 kJ

Photograph opposite (centre right)

Tip

This goes very well with boiled potatoes or a slice of buttered bread. Eaten with meat or fish, the vegetables provide a very satisfying protein meal.

MANGETOUT WITH CARROTS

Preparation time: 25 minutes

Serves 2

400 g/14 oz mangetout (sugar peas)
400 g/14 oz carrots
15 ml/1 tbsp butter
75 ml/3 fl oz/6½ tbsp water
10 ml/2 tsp vegetarian vegetable stock (instant powder)
5 ml/1 tsp honey
30 ml/2 tbsp finely chopped fresh parsley

1. Wash the mangetout and remove the side strips if necesssary.

2. Peel the carrots, rinse and dice.

3. Melt the butter in a saucepan. Add the mangetout and carrots and stir-fry for 7 minutes.

4. Add the water then season with vegetable stock and honey.

5. Cover the pan and simmer the vegetables slowly for 15 minutes. Serve sprinkled with parsley.

about 190 kcal/795 kJ

Photograph opposite (centre left)

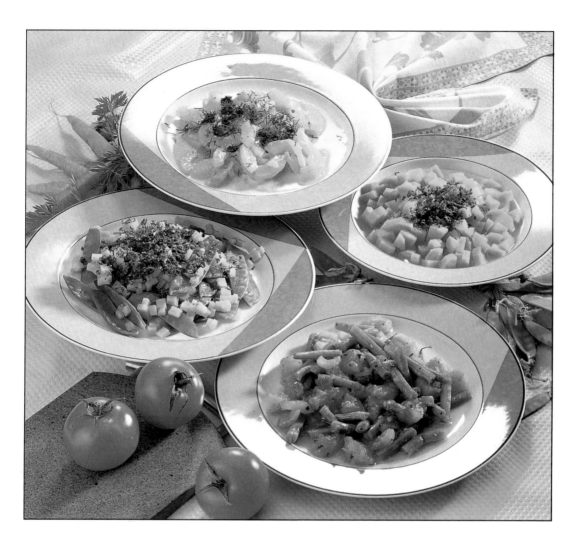

ITALIAN-STYLE GREEN BEANS

Preparation time: 35 minutes

Serves 2

450 g/1 lb green beans
sea salt
400 g/14 oz tomatoes
15 ml/1 tsp cold pressed olive oil
5 ml/1 tsp herb salt
10 ml/2 tsp crushed dried oregano
10 ml/2 tsp crushed dried rosemary

1. Wash the beans, remove the side strips if necessary and cut into 2.5/1 in pieces. Cook in lightly salted boiling water for about 10–15 minutes until *al dente*.

2. Blanch and skin the tomatoes then chop coarsely.

3. Heat the olive oil in a saucepan and add the tomatoes. Fry for 5 minutes, stirring. Drain the beans and add to the tomatoes. Season with herb salt, oregano and rosemary.

about 185 kcal/775 kJ

Photograph above (bottom)

POTATO PURÉE

Preparation time: 30 minutes

Serves 2

450 g/1 lb potatoes

300 ml/½ pt/1¼ cups boiling salted water

5 ml/1 tsp vegetarian vegetable stock (instant powder)

45 ml/3 tbsp single (light) cream

1. Peel and wash the potatoes. Cut into chunks and cook in boiling salted water until soft, keeping the pan half-covered.

2. Pour off half the cooking water then mash the potatoes in the remaining water. Beat until smooth and leave in the saucepan.

3. Season with vegetable stock and stir in the cream. Reheat over a low heat, whisking all the time.

about 230 kcal/960 kJ

Photograph opposite (top)

Tip

Baked onions and heated-up sauerkraut go well with the purée.

VINAIGRETTE DRESSING

Preparation time: 15 minutes

Serves 2

20 ml/4 tsp sunflower oil

5 ml/1 tsp herb salt

10 ml/2 tsp lemon juice

45 ml/3 tbsp water

1 large onion

30 ml/2 tbsp mixed chopped fresh herbs (parsley, chives, dill, mint, sorrel, tarragon, thyme, marjoram, borage and/or lemon balm)

1 clove garlic

1. Beat together the oil, herb salt and lemon juice. Thin down with water.

2. Peel the onion and garlic, chop finely and stir into the oil mixture with herbs.

about 110 kcal/460 kJ

Photograph opposite (centre)

Tip

This vinaigrette dressing goes well with all lettuce salads as well as salads made with steamed vegetables.

HERB SAUCE

Preparation time: 5 minutes

Serves 2

200 ml/7 fl oz/1 scant cup buttermilk

150 ml/¼ pt/⅔ cup soured (dairy sour) cream

100 g/4 oz mixed, chopped fresh herbs (parsley, sorrel, chervil, borage, cress, chives)

5 ml/1 tsp herb salt

10 ml/2 tsp lemon juice

1. Beat the buttermilk with the soured cream then mix in the herbs.

2. Season with herb salt and lemon juice.

about 140 kcal/590 kJ

Photograph opposite (bottom)

Tip

This herb sauce goes well with potatoes freshly boiled in their skins. It is also suitable as a dressing for salads and cooked vegetables.

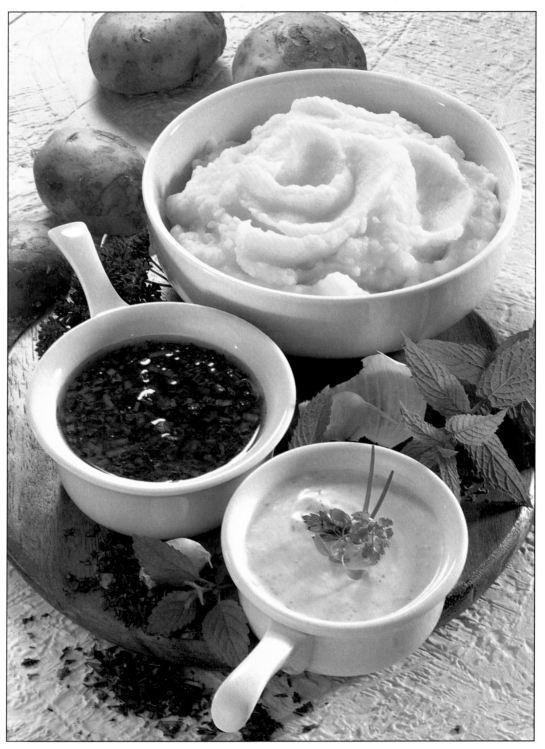

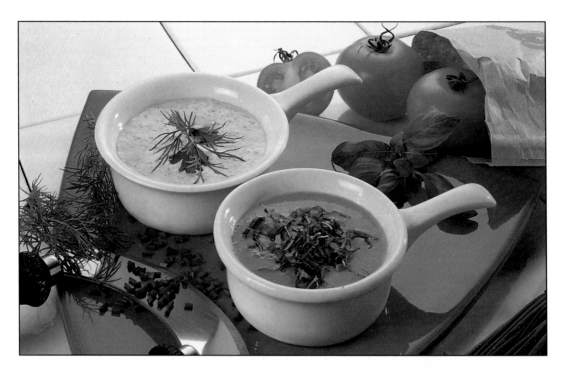

SPICY SALAD SAUCE

Preparation time: 10 minutes

Serves 2

175 ml/6 fl oz/¾ cup buttermilk or
  smetana

15 ml/1 tbsp lemon juice

5 ml/1 tsp herb salt

5 ml/1 tsp honey

100 ml/3½ fl oz/6½ tbsp water

10 ml/2 tsp sunflower oil

1 clove garlic

15 ml/1 tbsp chopped fresh herbs
  (parsley, dill, chives)

1. Beat together the buttermilk
or smetana, lemon juice, herb
salt and honey.

2. Stir in the water then whisk
in the oil.

3. Crush in the peeled garlic
then stir in the herbs.

about 180 kcal/750 kJ

Photograph above (left)

COLD TOMATO SAUCE

Preparation time: 10 minutes

Serves 2

400 g/14 oz tomatoes

150 ml/¼ pt/⅔ cup buttermilk or
  smetana

5 ml/1 tsp herb salt

1 large pinch of cayenne pepper

5 ml/1 tsp honey

10 ml/2 tsp chopped fresh basil

1. Blanch and skin the
tomatoes. Cut in quarters and
purée in a blender.

2. Whisk into the buttermilk or
smetana.

3. Season with herb salt,
cayenne pepper and honey.
Sprinkle with basil.

about 140 kcal/585 kJ

Photograph above (right)

Tip

This sauce goes very well with
raw vegetables.

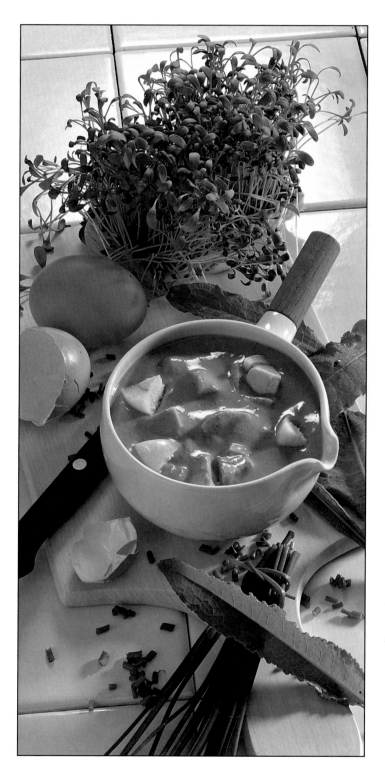

EGG AND HERB SAUCE

Preparation time: 15 minutes

Serves 2

100 g/4 oz mixed fresh herbs (sorrel, parsley, chervil, cress, chives, borage)
150 ml/¼ pt/⅔ cup buttermilk or smetana
150 ml/¼ pt/⅔ cup natural yoghurt, 3.5 per cent fat
5 ml/1 tsp herb salt

1. Hard boil the eggs. Shell when cold and chop.

2. Wash the herbs and shake dry. Put into blender with the buttermilk or smetana and yoghurt.

3. Season with herb salt then add eggs.

about 300 kcal/1255 kJ

Tip

This egg and herb sauce is suitable as a dressing for lettuce, raw vegetables and vegetable salads.

Recipe index